Shirley —
Change is everything!
All the best ☺ Lin

People Are Talking . . .

"The ideas you present in the ***7 Keys*** *are simple and real. They support the process of change as we make new choices in our lives. Most human beings don't like change, it is confusing and frightening. The help you provide through your book makes the change process more palatable!"*

— Judy Sabah, Business/Personal Coach, Professional Speaker, Co-founder/Past President, Colorado Speakers Association

"You brought an inspirational spark to our luncheon! We have gotten great feedback from our members. You gave many the gentle kick that you promised. Your experiences give your motivational talk backbone and credibility. Your enjoyment of the task pulls your audience up to the stage. You have a warm style that invites your listeners and readers to participate. The personal stories give your presentation texture, humor and relevancy.

You have a great story to share and the talents to share it vividly! You also made warm, personal connections with individuals you met prior to and after the luncheon. I have enjoyed your book as well. You give succinct insights into life. I am adopting the one phrase from your book — 'Live one day at a time and make it a masterpiece.'

Very few people live the theory of abundance. It's nice to meet a woman who embodies the theory in her actions. I would highly recommend you as a speaker to any organization looking to inspire and motivate its members. Thanks, Lin!"

— Keller Hayes, President, Colorado Women's Chamber of Commerce

"Just a note to thank you for your book. I've read it and am re-reading it. If I had to pick one point that spoke to me the most it would be living in the present moment. I live a lot in the past and worry about tomorrow. So, I'm practicing daily to live in this moment Right Now. WOW! An exciting new experience. Thanks again!"

— Wheatridge, CO

"I received your book. By just browsing through it I know I will absolutely love and definitely benefit from it. It's the type of book I will keep forever! Will read every word of it!"

— Spring Valley, NY

"Bravo for your new book!! I just finished reading it and I loved it. Having read about 250 books in psychology and spirituality over the past 11 years, I felt I had read it all. I couldn't imagine what you had to say that hadn't been said before. Your message is timely and one which I believe society is ready to hear. In concise, easy-to-read style, you give us the bottom line: no matter where we come from, no matter how dysfunctional our backgrounds, no matter what has happened to us along the way, ultimately we alone are responsible for making the necessary choices and changes in our lives to bring about lasting peace, joy, and healing."

— Golden, CO

"I loved it! I want to share it with friends!"

— Denver, CO

"I read your 7 Keys based on the acronym CHANGES. 'Hurt enough to want to change' Ouch! Well, you are exactly right. Pain is a great motivator. Since I moved here two years ago, life has been different. Some of those changes have been uncomfortable. I now understand that growth is nearly impossible without some level of discomfort.

I was very impressed by your Women's Forum presentation last year. I am sure to be equally inspired by your new book."

— Lakewood, CO

"I read 7 Keys and want to tell you how much I enjoyed it! Everything you have stated in the book is what we know, but so enlightening to see it in words and sentences!"

— Golden, CO

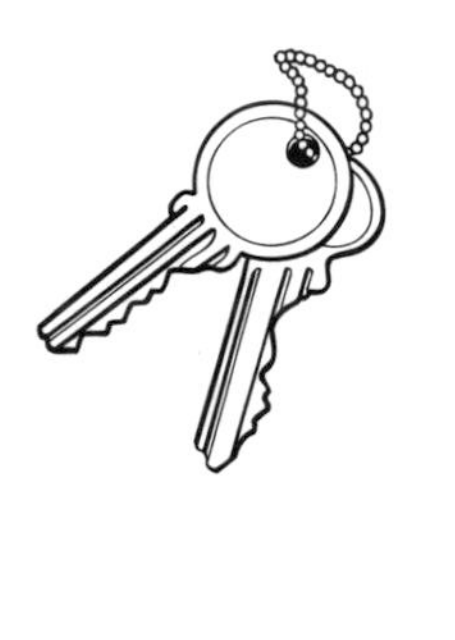

7 Keys to Changing

Your Life, Health and Wealth

by
Linda McNeil

Open Mind Publishing

First Edition

First Printing October, 1998

Manufactured in the United States of America

Cover and interior designer: Karen Saunders

Illustrator: Sean McCartney

Editor: Allison St. Claire

Library of Congress Catalog Card Number: 98-092010

ISBN 1-891446-02-9

Open Mind Publishing

P.O. Box 280234

Lakewood, CO 80228

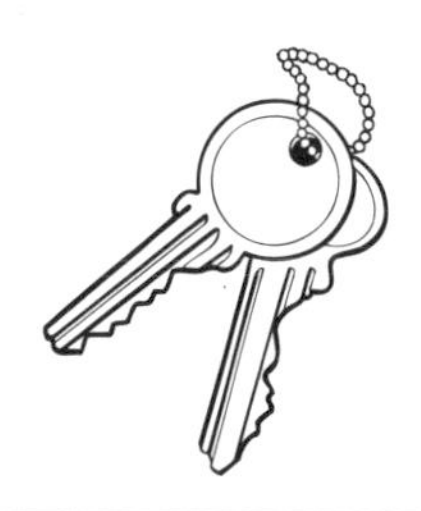

Table of Contents

In Gratitude:

Thank you, Maureen Christensen, for: your consistent encouragement, never doubting, always inspiring and supporting, unconditional love, and for "helping me keep my feet on the ground!"

Thank you, Cia Wenzel, for: being one of the most positive people I know, watching my finances, scuba diving, and always believing.

Thank you, Barbara Knapp-Colston, for: being a best friend since the 4th grade and always being there for me in love and companionship.

Thank you, Paul Williams, for: your very generous contributions to this book, for always being present and encouraging me to share my gifts.

I am grateful to you, Allison St. Claire, for being talented, dependable and also a fun and inspiring editor. You are a pleasure to work with!

Thank you, Mom and Dad, for: providing me a loving childhood and teaching me a deep appreciation of nature and the out-of-doors. You also taught me how to work hard—I've needed that!

I am grateful to you, Melissa Hubbell, for being my youngest best friend and teaching me more about play-time. I love you!

I am grateful to my brother, Randy, for getting my attention back in the beginning of this trip! Also, to his wife, Sandy, for her support and part in my abundant life.

I am thankful for all the people who purchased my first book and wrote letters, notes of gratitude, and especially to those have become friends.

Thank you to all the people whose stories I share with the reader, including Ken, Barb, Cia, Mom and Dad, and Paul.

Thank you to my new friend Jennifer Reinbrecht for sending me Sean McCartney, a talented illustrator, and to Karen Saunders, a skillful designer and valued member of the team.

Thank you to all the clients and seminar participants over the last ten years who have asked when I was going to write a book and reach beyond the limited arena of physical therapy. Here's to the big picture!

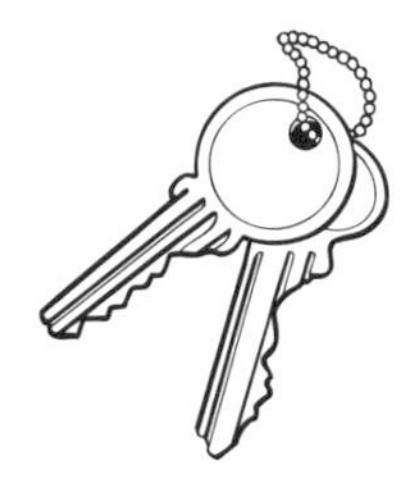

Introduction

I know change! You bet I do. And I know lots of other people who know change whose lives are miracles, too. How impossible it feels at times. How painful change can be. But how exciting!

How about you? Why did you pick up this book? I bet you know a little something about change yourself or you wouldn't have the book in your hands now. Either you want to change some aspect of your life, or you have to. You know that some part of your life isn't working, either personal or professional. You have begun to suspect that change is up to you — not the rest of the world, your boss, your spouse, your kids. So, you want to know how. What do you have to do?

What is my life experience that might convince you there are some ideas here that work? Well, 18 years ago I weighed 200 pounds and my blood pressure was 220/120. I am the only person I know who has lost one-third of her body weight and kept it off for 18 years. My blood pressure today is 120/60. I was told I would never be off blood pressure medication. I have been — since 1980.

I had more than a slight drinking and prescription drug problem. In fact, I am a 12+ years recovered alcoholic. Suffice it to say, I nearly lost a business and I did lose a marriage to my addictions. I even went to jail for a DUI and I greatly hurt most of the people in my life. I certainly hurt myself. In fact, I lost myself.

In the midst of all this, I had a seemingly successful physical therapy practice, although at one point in 1982 I went to an attorney to ask about the possibility of filing bankruptcy. You know what he said? "Put away your plastic and stop spending money you don't have!"

At another time I was in counseling with a wonderful man named Steve. I will never forget what he told me: "To change a habit, you must stop doing two things and start doing one."

He asked me how I went from the brink of bankruptcy to selling my physical therapy practice — which I started with $1100 insurance money from an automobile accident — to a public, national corporation after my business had reached yearly revenues of $1,200,000. The answer was simple in words, but hard to do. I stopped spending on credit, stopped being married to someone who spent like I did, and started taking responsibility for my fiscal future. Thank you, Steve. You were important in my life changes.

I am privileged to know people who got sober in prison. Many recovering people I know got so far down that they tried suicide as "the ultimate out." I did. I tried suicide three times. If I hadn't been married to my second spouse and he didn't know me better then I knew myself, I wouldn't be here to tell you about it.

Do I have it made now? Do I have all of life's answers? Absolutely not! I seem to project that image to people who hear me present at seminars, courses, and training sessions. But I am still learning. I know that at some level I have to keep growing — mentally, emotionally, spiritually. I am always seeking. The journey is the fun, and I hope it will always be an on-going process of growth. I never want to "arrive." That would mean the trip is over.

The decision to write this book — to move toward becoming a much more widely-known speaker, to build a speaking and writing empire — is one of the most difficult decisions I have made since the incredibly difficult one I made to sell my physical therapy practice. I find I am as much afraid of success (again?!) as of failure. I value my privacy very much, having been single for 16 years. I find that even when I do a seminar and people are excited and want more, I tend to pull back, go to my hotel room and assume an attitude of "I have given a few tools that work for me. Now it is your job to pick them up and try them out for yourself!" That attitude may have to change.

Do I have the energy and physical strength to give more? One thing is perfectly clear to me: I am on the planet to share talents granted to me by no merit of my own. I am here to serve.

It is my fervent hope that you will find something in this book to inspire you to change just one or two important areas in your life! They don't have to big things, maybe just small discomforts or habits. Or, perhaps you want to deal more effectively with imposed change.

The 7 Keys will help you either way. They will help you stay changed — if you are ready.

My purpose is to participate in huge transformation and change for me and anyone else who comes into my life. My mission is to help one million people change for the good. I invite you to now become one of those who will make this process your own.

The book is structured to inspire, motivate and then move you to action. You are invited to answer questions, do activities and write your own thoughts and commitments to change in all the white spaces.

Are you ready?

They must often change who would be constant in happiness or wisdom.

— Confucius

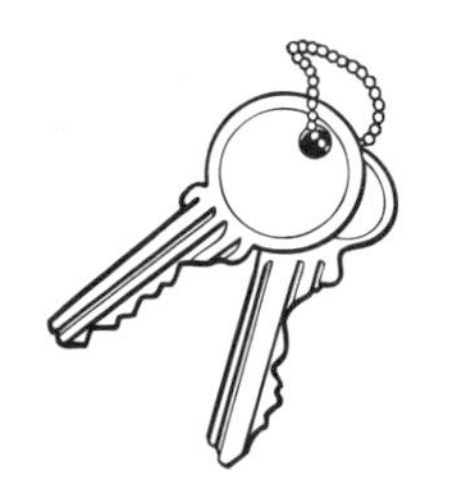

The Nature of Change

We seldom give much thought to change until our pain is intense, or change comes in the natural course of events, or we feel it is being forced upon us by no apparent choice of our own. What do we truly know about change?

There are two types: the change you opt for because you want to get a different result in some area of your life or there is imposed change over which you believe you have no control. Imposed changes might originate in the business from which you bring home a pay check. Those transitions might include mergers, acquisitions, downsizing, right-sizing, or any other "happening" on the job which seems to be not of your own choosing. These transformations can be extremely painful and I will not dwell on them here. This book is more for the types of changes you choose although it may also offer valuable clues to dealing with imposed change.

Change is inevitable. Until we breathe our last breath, change will continue. Something in our lives will always be evolving — body, mind, spirit, soul, society, the earth, the weather, technology, in other words, everything.

Some people have an easier time adapting to change than others. When I do team building with client companies and their employees, I frequently utilize a powerful personality profile called the DiSC™ Personal Profile System, from the

Carlson Learning Company in Minneapolis, Minnesota. This profile reveals each person's strengths, weaknesses, and tendencies under stress or when dealing with change. The profile helps clients and their employees see that change is very individual, and how each person adapts to change in his or her own way and time. The general traits and tendencies apply both personally and professionally.

Following are the four basic types of personalities:

- **Dominant** personalities' main characteristic is dominance; they demand, dominate, have high ego-strength, are goal oriented, impatient and motivated by challenges. They make things happen! Their basic fears are being taken advantage of and loss of control. They crave and need change, like lifeblood. They don't always consider all the ramifications of change, therefore their course is frequently not well thought out and does not always bring the best results. Under pressure and during times of change, they may show lack of concern for others' views and feelings.

- **Inducers/Influencers** are very optimistic. They are motivated by social recognition and lots of people contact. They utilize their considerable verbal and communication skills to negotiate just about everything. Their basic fear is social rejection. They also love change. They need it, thrive upon it, and are a lot more people-oriented than task-oriented. Their approach is very team-driven, along the lines of "Come on, team, *we* can do it." During times of change and when under pressure influencers can become quite disorganized and unfocused.

- **Steadiers** are very patient, easy-does-it personalities, who are a little more laid back than the two previous types. They are very team oriented and are consistent performers. Steadiers are motivated by the status quo, so they are not particularly fond of change. In fact, their basic fear is loss of stability or change. Steadiers need a lot of time and information ahead of time to process how change will affect them and their jobs. They will accept transition if they have time, information, and can see reason(s) to change. When change is imminent or when these people are under pressure, they can become overly willing to give. Steadiers have a hard time saying "no."

- **Conscientious** people are very analytical, task-oriented and show a lot of attention to details. They are highly motivated by correctness and quality. Their basic fear is criticism of their work, or not being able to do their jobs perfectly. Therefore, they like change the least of all four styles. Because they have a serious need to handle details and their jobs correctly, change greatly threatens their status quo, sense of security and control. They need a lot of guidance and detailed information about why and how in order to handle transition. It is helpful to involve them in the decision-making process, when and where change is necessary so that they have a vested interest in the results. During times of change or when under pressure, they can become overly critical of self and others.

Most stress indices assign high points for losses and even for changes that most people consider positive, such as marriage or moving to a better place. There is still stress associated with loss of the old, familiar way.

Most of us did not learn much about the mechanics of change at home or in school. Therefore, we are pretty uncomfortable with change and don't necessarily know how to alter behaviors, or make transitions positively and creatively. When I was in college, there were no courses on adapting to our changing world or creating new behaviors for increased success.

Fear is a typical initial reaction to the idea of change, whether imposed by or from an outside source, or through your own choice. What do we fear?

Most of us fear the unknown. I believe that if we took all our troubles and piled them in front of us, then went wandering around the planet seeking to take over someone else's preferably smaller pile, we eventually would come back to our own pile of troubles because we already know how to do them! We are familiar with our own problems and life issues. The unfamiliar is more scary and uncomfortable than what we already know.

We cannot change anyone else. Unfortunately, many of us spend much of our lives waiting for someone else to change so we will be happier, richer, have more freedom, or whatever. We truly would prefer that the rest of the world change first! We may think we can change others, but we can't.

In my seminar "Management by 100% Responsibility," I ask participants if they have ever been able to change another human being. Once in a while I get a young newlywed or other relationship neophyte who truly believes s/he has changed the new partner. What is revealed is that another person only changes when s/he chooses to change — ideas, behaviors, whatever — to his or her own benefit, and when and how s/he decides to internalize it for self. We cannot change anyone but ourselves.

Do you want to change the behavior of someone in your life? Have you already tried and failed? You can, indeed, make it worthwhile for another person to change — when you are willing to change yourself at the same time. This technique is called modeling and it works like this: If you want the other person to be punctual, model that behavior by being on time yourself. Explain why it is important to you to be prompt and to have the other person also be on time. Request that he or she also value being on time and consider doing so. Chances are pretty good the other person will decide to try that new behavior. But you cannot make the person do it. You can only set an example, lead the way, and request that the other person follow your example.

To me, being on time for an appointment demonstrates respect for the other person. His or her time is as important as mine is to me. It is a matter of honesty, integrity, intention, and keeping my word.

I had a friend whose time always seemed much more important than mine (and I charge well for mine!). She was constantly 30 to 45 minutes late. My value system doesn't tolerate that. She chose not to change. She could have started earlier; returned that last phone call later; respected my time. I ended the relationship.

Parents often think they can change their children and often spend huge amounts of time and energy trying to do so — usually futilely. They use both bribes and threats to a child to modify his or her behavior. However, if the child's change is not an internal and personal choice, the child will only perform the "good" behavior when the parent is still watching, and is still bigger and more powerful than the child. The new behavior will last only when the internal motivation is strong and positive enough. The child initiates and persists in a new behavior out of personal motivation and need.

We admire people who truly change their lives and keep them changed! We love stories about "winners" who turn their lives around, do something seemingly impossible or heroic — such as overcoming an addiction, recovering from cancer, or triumphing in spite of very difficult circumstances.

Truly effective and long-lasting change never comes from outside of self. Change is an inside job. Someone else may make it worthwhile by saying: "Change or lose your job," "Change or I will leave the marriage." But true change can only be internal and your own individual choice.

Real change is possible and can be forever. I am always saddened when I hear someone make the statement that nothing can truly change, that real change is impossible or that it cannot be lasting. Well, those statements are wrong. If you have them in your thinking, push them out. I am proof of lasting change in numerous areas. I know many people whose changes have been major, real and have lasted for many, many years. The 7 Keys are offered as tools to help you make real, lasting "altered behaviors."

The one thing you can always choose is your attitude. The one thing you can always change is your attitude!

What do you want to change in your life? Your health, body, wealth? A circumstance, belief, attitude, situation? Are you ready to examine the hows and whys of change? If you are, read the following nine chapters with your hearts and minds wide open and discover how to make your new choices into effective, lasting life changes.

I do not have all the answers. I don't even know all the questions. However, I have had much experience with choices and changes that have empowered me in ways I never even imagined. May you also be empowered!

What we know about change:

- There are two types of change: chosen and imposed.
- Change is inevitable.
- Some people adapt to change easier than others.
- Even people who love change can be stressed after a point.
- Most of us didn't learn how to do change in early life.
- Fear is a typical reaction to change.
- We cannot change anyone else.
- We admire people who truly change and stay changed.
- Effective change is an inside job.
- Real change is possible and can be forever.

To pretend to change anyone is an illusion: he picks up his first trail at the first occasion.

— La Fontaine

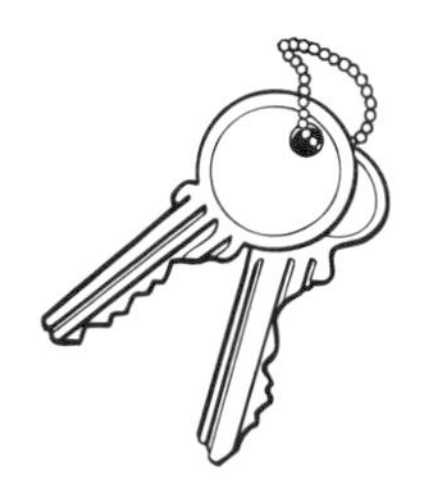

Key # 1:

Choose Differently

For Key #1 — choose differently — to begin to work for us, we first must deal with the issue of choice. When I was fat, there were many mornings I got up and decided "This is the day! I don't want to be size 22 any longer. I hate myself this way."

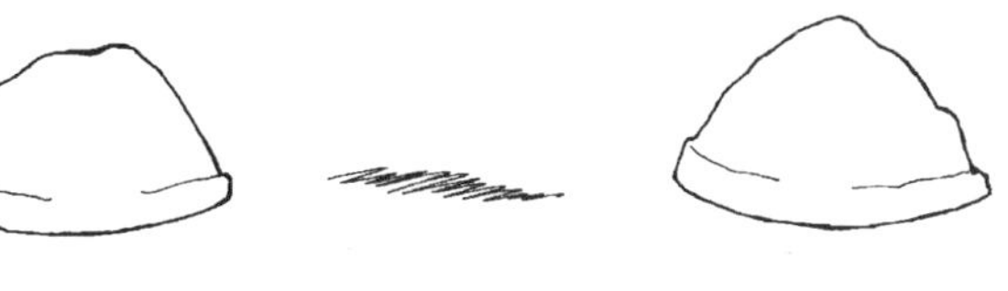

I have been on more types of diets than I can remember. I even tried that awful liquid protein diet that killed people in the 1970's by making their hearts go electrically haywire! At the time, I didn't realize that I chose to be fat. It wasn't a conscious or knowing choice.

What is the magical turning point? When do you arrive at the day when you really mean you are ready for change — you know that this is truly the bottom of the barrel? Webster's Dictionary defines change as "shift, movement, transformation, transition, alter, make different." When does your transition truly begin?

If you are being abused, hopefully you arrive at a realization like this: "I am out of excuses for leaving . . . for believing if I act differently s/he will react differently. I deserve better." You choose to do whatever it will take to obtain a different result, a better result. You decide. You understand you are choosing to be where you are.

If you are angry and negative and want to be more positive and peaceful, one day you say, "I am not happy. This is not a good way to spend the short days of my life. This is my life and I don't want to live it like this any more!" You then are choosing a different way.

If you have been blaming your family, the past, the government, the boss, the kids, the weather, whatever, for all your misery and problems, one day you look around and see someone who is happy and taking charge of the results in his or her life. Bingo! You get it. That's it. Time to move on. Time to let go. Time to forgive. You are choosing a different way.

Only you know when you have had enough of your problem. Only you can decide to choose a different way. Choice is hard. Too bad that it has to come first, because a lot of people give up right here. You've got to want to change so much it consumes you. So, get it out of the way. Make choices now. It works like this:

Webster's Dictionary says 'Choose' is: "opt for, select, decide, pick, take one thing in preference to another." 'Choice' is: "opportunity of choosing, selection."

Abraham Lincoln said, "Most people are about as happy as they make up their minds to be."

I say my life is easy for me when everything is working: my professional life is productive, my marriage is satisfying and solid, my finances are doing well, investments are earning a good return. I say, "Yes, I made these choices. I am proud of them. I accept the credit. I'd like a raise, pat on the back, my own private office. Yes, I did that. I will happily take the credit for my choices. I made great choices!"

However, when the marriage falls apart, I am being abused, I am sick, miserable, broke, addicted, angry, resentful, in jail, my first reaction is: "It's not my fault! It's yours, his, hers, Mom's, Dad's, the IRS, the ex-wife, the past, the future, the boss, God, Satan, the government, the kids . . . ad infinitum."

It seems to be human nature to blame others. In addition, our litigious culture has taught us that nothing is our fault. Or, in some families, maybe we were taught that everything is our fault, in which case we probably still were not taught the difference among fault and blame and/or responsibility.

To choose does not necessarily mean to wish or want. It just means choose. Choosing doesn't mean knowing with absolute clarity or with full information.

For instance, if I choose to smoke, it definitely is a choice. No one else is making me smoke. I decide to buy the cigarettes, then I smoke them. I probably do that because I am cool, I think smoking is cool, I want to fit in and I believe I am infallible and that I will be the one never to get lung cancer or emphysema or chronic obstructive pulmonary disease.

Victim? Accident? Bad luck?

No. Choice. A casually made choice, without any results in mind except the rewards of the moment. So, I choose to smoke, not necessarily wishing, wanting, or knowing whether it will cause cancer.

Where is the choice in divorce if you want to keep your marriage and your partner wants to end it? Obviously, your first choice was to get married. Even if there was a factor like pregnancy, you still had other choices and alternatives. With any other personal relationship, there are always many possibilities. The problem is most of us have been taught one way to think, to do, to view what is "right." Therefore, we don't recognize all of our choices.

Sometimes we do not know what our choices are until we get clear on the concept that we have choices. Other times we choose unknowingly. It is important to leave out blame, shame and guilt.

Did you know that "right" isn't an absolute concept? Right is merely what I say that you agree with. Somebody else hears me and it is wrong to them, based on their set of life experiences, learned values, and beliefs.

Possibly you were brought up in a church that taught you their way absolutely is the only "right" way. Your church and my church may have used the same Book but concluded something totally different from its contents; that is, "Our way is the only 'right' way! You don't do things this way, you will go to hell, be punished, or burn, or whatever." Can we all be absolutely "right" — using the same book? Or is it a matter of "right" being what you were taught?

Let's get back to the marriage that is falling apart. The initial choice (either conscious or unconscious) was to get married or not to get married. Then there was a series of choices (conscious or unconscious): stay married or not, be happy or unhappy; be faithful or unfaithful (we don't just happen into affairs), go to counselling or not, go to church or not, have children or not, etc. One of the frightening things in our society is that we seem to think these things just sort of happen to us. It is not that way. We make choices.

How about some of the really tough issues? Do we choose abuse or disease? Or are we victims of a sick society, an evil world, a dysfunctional family? Does terminal illness just happen to us, or is it the fault of our parents, our genetics? Remember, choosing does not necessarily mean wishing or wanting, it simply means choosing.

Does the child with leukemia choose the disease? How can a child choose abuse? There are people that you and I know who believe in truly 100% responsibility; they believe in the concept of reincarnation and, therefore, believe that they even choose their parents for a lesson to be learned in this lifetime.

I haven't arrived at that understanding, but I try to keep my mind open. I do know there are times when it seems disease just "happens" by no act of our own. When I get really honest, I can see some of the choices that may have contributed to the underlying or even active causes thereof. They may have been knowing or unknowing choices, consciously or unconsciously made.

Even if true victimization does exist and the world truly is a terrible place, or God is a vengeful god or the Devil plays dirty tricks on us, even if we cannot get to an analytical understanding of causes and choices, we are left with the choices that make up our lives after the horrible happening or victimization (or even the imposed business event we talked about earlier).

If you were sexually or physically abused, at what point are you willing to choose your reaction differently and stop allowing victimization to continue affecting and determining your happiness or unhappiness today?

If you are dealing with a terminal disease, what are the choices facing you today? I am not saying you got up one day, decided your life was a bit boring and said, "I think I will choose cancer." I am saying you might have chosen certain high-risk behaviors that put you in a position to not do all it takes to protect yourself against cancer.

You may not agree or even understand all I've said about choice. My intention here is to upset your usual way of seeing the world! I invite you out of your "brain-box" and to open your mind to seeing things in a different way!

I know this. I chose to be fat. I chose to drink. I chose to abuse drugs and my body. I chose to spend in a totally irresponsible manner. No one ever forced me to eat, drink, take drugs or spend all the money I earned, plus more. Now I choose to eat well, not drink, not drug and demonstrate good stewardship of money. Life is different. It is better. So are the results.

Is it easy? Now it is. Choice was not an easy concept in the beginning, however. Plus, new habits and behaviors take practice and more practice.

If you have a terminal disease and can't see that you made any choices to cause it, all that matters now is the series of choices you are currently making to deal with this reality. I am not saying that if you have an advanced case of cancer, you can just now decide to not have it. In a most real sense, that could be dangerous denial. However, there are people who believe that the mind is so powerful as to be able to heal anything, with the help of a Higher Power, and a whole lot of spiritual work.

101 Choices We All Make

1. Who we are
2. Who we love
3. Who we become
4. Who we help
5. Who we hang out with
6. Who we work with
7. Who we play with
8. Who we work for
9. Who we travel with
10. Who we support
11. Who we listen to
12. Who we share ourselves with
13. Who we marry
14. Who we don't marry
15. Who we have as friends
16. What we do with our lives
17. What career(s) we choose
18. What job(s) we take

19. What we are
20. What we love
21. What we love to do
22. What we think
23. What we spend our time on
24. What we believe in
25. What our lives look like
26. What we relate to
27. What we put in our minds
28. What we read
29. What we watch on television
30. What we listen to
31. What we feel
32. What we participate in
33. What we contribute to
34. When we grow up
35. When we leave the past behind
36. When we marry
37. When we work
38. When we play
39. When we love
40. When we hate
41. When we are happy
42. When we are unhappy

43. When we participate in life
44. When we don't participate in life
45. When we do anything
46. When we think good thoughts
47. When we think bad thoughts
48. Where we live
49. Where we don't live
50. Where we play
51. Where we work
52. Where we travel
53. Where we don't travel
54. Where we do anything
55. Why we love
56. Why we hate
57. Why we do or choose any of the above
58. Why we think the thoughts we think
59. Why we work
60. Why we play
61. How we work
62. How we play
63. How we make love
64. How we love
65. How we express ourselves
66. How we grow spiritually
67. How we don't grow spiritually
68. How we think

69. How we dress
70. How we drive
71. How we look
72. How we do sports
73. How we participate in life
74. How we don't participate in life
75. How we do friendship
76. How we share
77. How we don't share
78. How happy we are
79. How unhappy we are
80. How friendly we are
81. How courteous we are
82. How angry we are
83. How peaceful we are
84. How much we share
85. How much we make
86. How much we travel
87. How much we love
88. How much we contribute
89. How much we work
90. How much we play
91. How much we know
92. How much we don't know
93. How much we care
94. How much we live

95. How much we die
96. How much we want
97. How much we are grateful for
98. How much we are willing to do
99. How much we are willing to give
100. How much we believe in something
101. How much of a difference we make in our lifetime.

Choose Differently:

- We choose all our current realities.
- If they are good, we're willing to take credit for them.
- If they are bad, we tend to blame others.
- To get different results and to move forward (change) we must choose differently.
- There are at least 101 choices we each make.

You don't get to choose how you're going to die or when. You can only decide how you're going to live.

— Joan Baez

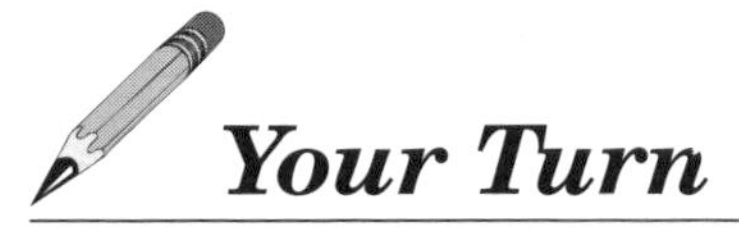

Your Turn

1. What are all the choices that got me where I am today?

2. What results do I want to create?

Destiny is not a matter of chance, it is a matter of choice; it is not a thing to be waited for, it is a thing to be achieved.

— William Jennings Bryan

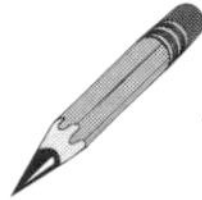

Your Turn

3. What are different choices I need to make now to create the results I want?

Are you hearing a lot of "Yeah, but's . . ." in your head as you write? You know, "Yeah, but I didn't choose that!" Try this technique. Every time you hear yourself saying "Yeah, but . . .," stop. Ask what choices you made. Ask what your part was in the final result. Then what choices you need/want to make. This is not about shame or blame — only an altered perspective. Keep writing.

The best way out of a difficulty is through it.

— Anonymous

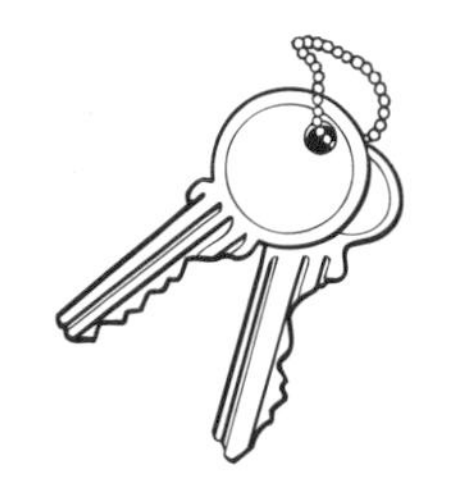

Key # 2:

Hurt Enough to Want to Change

There all types of pain — physical, mental, spiritual, social. If any part of your life is miserable or painful enough, at some point you come to recognize the pain as something you are not willing to live with anymore. Then you begin to choose differently.

When I drank, I would get up in the morning and decide not to drink, or only have one at lunch, or two or four at "twofers-time." Or I would decide to diet and not drink at lunch. I was a terrible liar. I never did what I said. Once I started, I couldn't stop or control the amount I drank. It was pretty much the same with food, pills and spending. My behavior was crazy. I hurt myself and others. I went to jail. Yet, the outside world

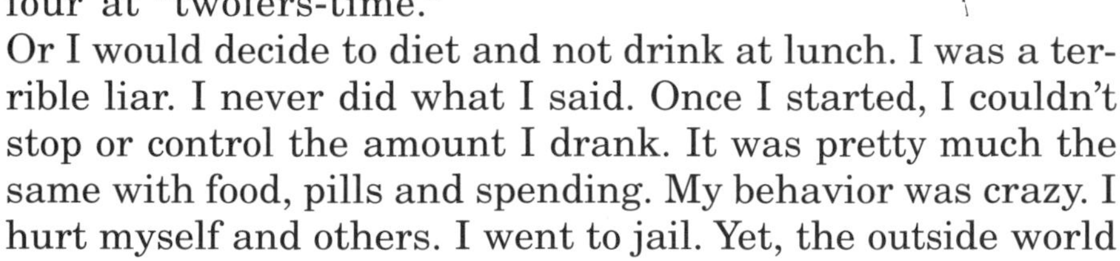

saw a "successful" woman, owner of a small business, with all the "trappings" of success.

Let's look at the other side of those trappings — and they were indeed traps!

> *As all these behavior patterns continued to progress, thoughts of suicide seemed to take me over more and more frequently, especially during long winter evenings at home. Despite all the beautiful areas in our house, I huddled on the floor of the bathroom next to the kitchen where I would lock myself in with the telephone.*
>
> *The more I drank, the more depressed I became and the more impossible everything seemed. I had already been hospitalized for depression once. No one had been able to impress upon my softening, drug and alcohol-soaked brain, that alcohol is a depressant. So, depressed I was. I hated my body. I was angry at the world. I hated myself.*
>
> *One time while locked in the bathroom I had a conversation with my mother about my weight and sunk into the deepest morass of self-pity. I not only hated myself, but I was going to show her! I would just kill myself.*
>
> *Cowered in the corner, I sobbingly wrote the most pathetic of suicide notes. I still have it. Why do I still keep fat pictures and such things as suicide notes around? To remember how bad it was so I never go back there. To remember that I hurt enough to want to change.*
>
> *My husband finally gave up on coaxing me out into the land of the living.*
>
> *Frequently these long crying sessions would lead to my calling suicide hot lines to ask for*

> *help and tell them how bad I had it. If they had only known! I am pretty sure they must have told me to go get help for the drinking and sober up! But I just don't remember.*
>
> *Blackouts had now become a regular problem. Blackouts are an incredibly frightening phenomenon of addiction. One time I actually signed business loan papers in a blackout. That means later I had absolutely no recall of having been there or done that. When in a drug or alcohol induced blackout, a person can appear, talk and function in an apparently normal fashion. I didn't know I was in a blackout and no one else had any way of knowing either. Eventually, I just ended up with all these holes in time. They were long and short periods of time I can not account for and of which I have no memory. At times certain people seemed to think I had blackouts for convenience sake.*
>
> *Then paranoia truly set in, followed by the sucking, black abyss of depression once again.*

As my weight was quickly increasing, I hated shopping for clothes. Nothing old fit and nothing new appealed. My feelings of disgust with myself increased every time I had to look in the mirror or try to figure out what to wear. I was embarrassed and humiliated.

When I was shopping or eating out, I thought I knew what everyone else was thinking about my gross body. Often I would not even try clothes on in the store. It felt less conspicuous if I just guessed at the size, grabbed something from the rack, paid for it and went home.

One time my husband was shopping with me when I decided to go ahead and try on the clothes I wanted to buy. I shyly came out of the dressing room to show them to him. As

I walked back into the cubicle, I overhead the clerk say to my husband, "Your wife has the most beautiful face."

I wanted to die, even though what she said was probably meant to be a lovely compliment. To me it meant everything else. Shame was taking over my thinking.

Some time later I read a book called "I'm Dancing As Fast As I Can" (Harper & Row, NY, 1979), written by Barbara Gordon, an award-winning television producer. Ms. Gordon got hooked on legally prescribed Valium, then tried to get herself off the medication, without a doctor or hospitalization. Withdrawal from Valium without help can be deadly. I was impressed by a similar scenario in her book when she needed a fancy dress for a special occasion and was too crazy and self-conscious to take the time to try it on. She ran in the store, grabbed something off the rack, paid for it and fled for home. After that she tried her best to get it together and appear "normal" for the important event.

And I thought I was the only one!

> *Here is my personal "hitting-bottom" story: January, 1980. I got on the scales, and tipped it at 200 pounds. I am five feet four. That means I was wearing size 22. I was fat. My brother was getting married and I had a very hard time finding a petite, fat dress for the wedding. I still carry a picture of me sitting at the wedding. (You can see it on the back cover of this book). As you can see, I did not look very happy.*
>
> *My then-husband and I lived in a big, four-bedroom house on a hill. We had a large yard, waterfalls, and lovely pools. The house was furnished well. From the outside, it looked as though we had the perfect life. We had snow-mobiles, motorcycles, and numerous expensive toys. I drove a champagne-gold, jazzy little Datsun 280ZX.*

I tried suicide three times. I hated myself. My business was struggling (it got worse later!); I had 35 employees whose children I worried about feeding. My marriage was just a marriage — not necessarily happy, not necessarily unhappy. My husband did just about anything to keep me and the lifestyle going. We spent a lot of money — eating out at night, drinking, playing, generally living the "high" life and impressing others. We had no savings and no investments. We spent it all.

On that day in January 1980 when I got on the scales, and saw 200 pounds, I also looked in the mirror and actually saw my red eyes, broken blood vessels on my cheeks, the horrible gray pewter color of my skin.

"What the hell is wrong with you?" I snarled. "You have everything. I hate you. I hate my body. I hate myself." I couldn't seem to die, and I couldn't seem to live. I suddenly knew I needed help.

As my husband and I sat down to lunch that day with my sister-in-law, I said quietly, "I think I'm an alcoholic. I need help." My husband nearly fell off his chair. (As though he didn't know).

My sister-in-law said, "That's the best news I've heard in a long time. I hope you know your family loves you very much and will stand by you no matter what."

What a miracle! And they did, to the best of their ability and understanding of what we all came to know as the disease of alcoholism.

I used to go to the doctor a lot, and to the hospital at least yearly, whether I needed it or not. When I showed up that day, his nurse said, "What is it this time, Lin?"

The doctor got right to work and had me admitted as soon as possible. Thus began one of the most amazing and challenging journeys of my life. I would not trade it for all the gold on the planet. I have witnessed many miracles and mine is just one of the small ones. Getting off pills and losing weight at the same time I quit drinking was a major challenge — and typically not medically advisable. I am very lucky to be alive.

I only know that for me I reached enough pain. My clothes didn't fit. The three suicide attempts didn't work. The lonely space in my head was expanding. The hole in my soul was so big there wasn't enough of anything to fill it. I suspected that I had "hit bottom" and I hurt enough to want to change.

Hitting bottom can apply to anything — mental or emotional state of mind, physical condition, spiritual condition, drinking, drugging, abuse, etc. Others might think they are being helpful when they try to get you to deal with an obvious problem, but until the pain is great enough, you do not recognize the "bottom."

With addictions, it is said that sometimes the bottom rises up to meet you. Some people lose everything — family, home, job(s), self-respect, money, stability, possessions, perhaps go to prison or a mental health institution — before they "hit bottom." Some die. No one else can determine how low "bottom" is.

Other people choose to get off the sinking elevator before it reaches the basement. The pain might be enough when something relatively minor happens. Perhaps the boss notices a botched job, or the spouse relates an embarrassing incident, or a blackout gets the person in trouble or just scares him. Or the person may see the bottom coming when the doctor says, "Quit smoking, quit drinking, lose weight or you're going to die." Only the person with the pain knows when he or she has hit bottom.

A 40-something male friend of mine was having some physical problems and went to a doctor. The diagnosis was diabetes. He had been drinking heavily, was overweight, and was having other difficulties. I asked my friend how he was able to simply make a decision, then do it. I really wanted to know if he was at his "bottom."

He said that when the doctor told him his diabetes could be treated with daily medication, change of diet, weight loss and exercise, it became instantly clear to him that if he wanted to stay alive, he must comply. His most meaningful motivator was the desire to watch his kids grow up and to be part of their lives. Amazingly, he stopped drinking, lost weight, began playing golf and working out on a regular basis. Today, he looks and feels entirely different.

That tells me he had not yet crossed the invisible line from casual or social drinking into the disease of alcoholism. Many alcoholics, when told by their doctors that they absolutely cannot take another drink or they will die, simply still cannot stop drinking. They have not yet reached a sufficiently painful "bottom." Certainly in some instances, the doctor telling an alcoholic "Stop or die" may be their hitting bottom. The point is: No one else can decide when you have had enough pain. Only you know.

If "hurt enough to want to change" does not make sense to you yet, you have not reached the limit of your pain — and you may not be ready to change.

> *About six months before I realized I had hurt enough, my brother, Randy, was visiting our home. I was fat, angry and drinking, as usual.*
>
> *He said, "I am going to say something to you which is probably going to make you really mad! You are going to call me names and very likely order me out of your home. But, that is a risk I am just going to have to take. What is it*

> *with you? How can you live in this beautiful home with a wonderful husband and be doing what you are doing to yourself? Every time I see you, you have a drink in your hand! What is the matter with you?"*
>
> *I immediately did exactly as he predicted: called him a lot of nasty names and ordered him out of our home! I don't even remember what happened next. However, I do know that although I did not respond immediately by quitting all my self-destructive behaviors, it must have gotten my attention at some level. I have never forgotten it, and I did make big decisions and choices within months of that conversation.*

My loving brother couldn't make me hurt enough to change in his time frame, but he could get my attention and let me know he cared. I am very grateful he cared enough to take that risk. When I was privileged to observe my tenth year sober, he came to the party to share in the celebration! Is that cool, or what?

If you understand "hurt enough" and you are in enough pain that you really want to change, you are well on your way. You have a serious need or desire to change.

How can you know for sure that you are ready? Go back to your old behavior. If the pain returns in sufficient force, you can be assured it is not going to disappear on its own. You must help it disappear.

A woman friend of mine decided to lose weight, for real. I had watched her doing what I did over and over: go on a diet, exercise, lose weight, gain it back; go on a diet, exercise, lose weight, gain it back. I asked her what made her finally decide to go to Weight Watchers and lose 35 pounds. She said she "hit bottom" one day when she bent over to tie her shoe laces and could hardly reach them. Her emotional pain was strong enough that the magic happened. "This is it!" she declared.

I admire her very much. Since Weight Watchers, she has kept off most of the weight; she is now a competitive bicycle rider. She rides for charities and she maintains a highly successful career as a stock broker. She is my broker, in fact, for which I am very fortunate and grateful.

The 7 Keys in this book will also work for less drastic and obvious choices to change. Not all changes need be as dramatic as that of addicts — because not everyone has to hurt that bad. The point is that if people in dire straits can do amazing about-faces, you certainly can use these Keys to change habits like perfectionism, being late, constant criticism, anger, being judgmental, feeling disgusted or unhappy with your life.

If there is a behavior pattern in your relationships which you have tried to change and you know it costs you friendships, you may experience sufficient discomfort to get serious about wanting to change. Many people have a serious desire to be involved in a romantic relationship. They will get into one and are madly in love for several months while everything is perfect, dreamy, and idealistic. Then they start seeing all kinds of things wrong with the other not-so-perfect person. They begin criticizing. The other person, who began as lovely and nurturing now is like a totally different person.

What happened? How can you change such a problem? How can you change resistance to a truly intimate and whole relationship? Beginning to change the pattern is being willing to launch the next "Key." Ask for help and accept responsibility for your choices.

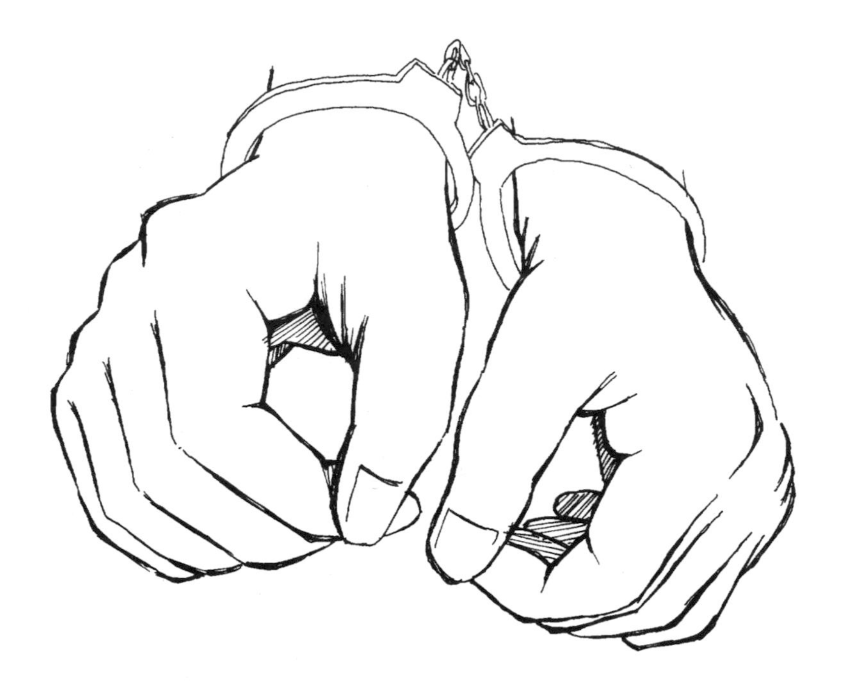

Change your choices —
Change your life!

Hurt enough to want to change:

- Change is painful so unless there's something painful enough to cause us to want to, most of us won't.
- No one else can cause us to hurt enough to change.
- I had to hit bottom in four different areas, all major. You may have multiple needs, too.
- Hitting bottom need not be relative to only big issues, but can also apply to smaller behavior changes.
- You are the only one who knows if you are ready to change, major or minor ways of being, doing, living, or thinking.

Others can stop you temporarily, only you can do it permanently.

— Dr. Robert Anthony

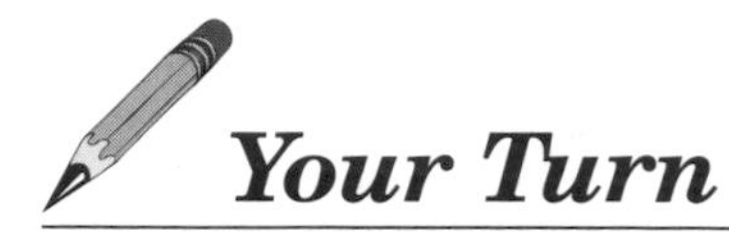

Your Turn

1. Where in my life do I feel pain — from physical symptoms like headaches to painful feelings like shame or guilt?

2. Is the pain sufficient enough to motivate me to change — to make different choices?

The pain of the mind is worse than the pain of the body.

— Syrus

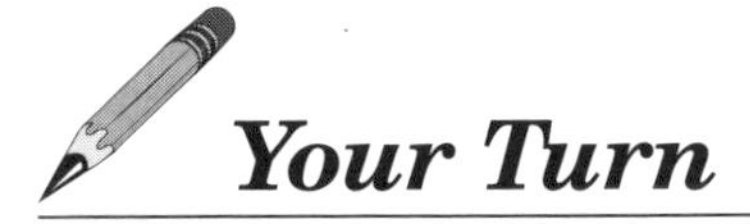

Your Turn

3. What will my life be like without hurting? Will I be: Sober? Thin? Happy? Without abuse? Financially stable?

4. Do I really want life without pain? What will I be like when I am truly free to live fully and joyfully?

The pain passes
but the beauty remains.

— Pierre Auguste Renoir

Key # 3:

Ask for Help and Accept Responsibility for Your Choices

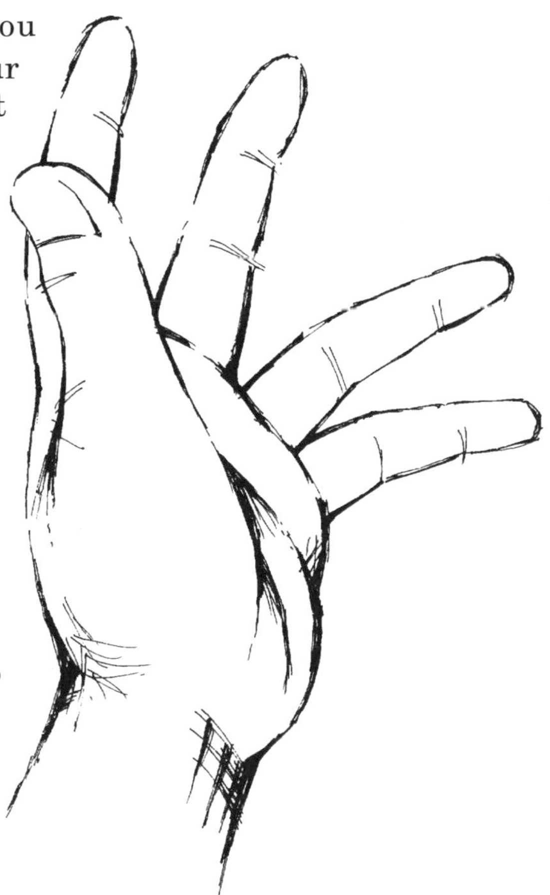

No matter what you want to change in your life — something that has cost you, caused some difficulty or pain — someone has been there before you! Someone has written a book. Or there is a self-help group. Or your neighbor knows someone who has been just about where you are. Or you might want to seek the help of a professional counselor. There is already a vast body of knowledge to help you change in a positive way.

What do you think is the hardest thing about deciding to

change? I think sometimes it is the feeling that you are uniquely alone. The feeling that no one else has been in exactly your same circumstances or has your past history or a similar problem. This belief alienates you from the help you want and can find. You find yourself terribly alone deep in your heart. Asking for help is absolutely essential to begin the mechanics of change.

- Asking for help is humbling. That's a good starting place to build a healthy self-esteem.
- Asking for help creates a connection to others who have been down the path before you. Relatedness is necessary for mutual support and information-sharing. You can learn what to do.
- Asking for help opens your eyes and ears, maybe even your heart and mind.
- Asking for help gets you out of the squirrel cage of your own thinking.

Is weight loss your goal? First, admit to your innermost self that you are fat, that you indeed need help. That is humbling. That is a beginning.

Next, go to a support group, such as Weight Watchers. They have a great reputation for helping thousands of people turn their lives around. On arrival, you'll see many people of all sizes, shapes and places of progress in their weight loss. Some are at the beginning — just like you. Many are much fatter. Some don't even look like they belong there. (They are the ones returning to check in, to remember what they were, and to what they will return if they don't remain vigilant).

The other fat members rush to share their stories with you. They have learned that they make more progress by sharing their experiences, strength, and hope. That is why you're there. By listening, you learn what to do, how long it takes to change your habits. What will it feel like when you actually see the new thin, real you emerge? How will you look? How will others react to you? Will you like the new you?

I can answer that question fairly accurately. When I was losing my first 40 pounds in 1980, I spent several months in the San Diego, California area, on the "island" of Coronado. I was totally unprepared for the need for my mind to catch up to my body.

> *My brain and my body never seemed to get together — to be in the same place at the same time! I'd been drinking heavily for eight years. I'd been gaining and losing weight since age 13 but most of my weight gain and dangerously elevated blood pressure took place in the same eight years as my drinking. In fact, the weight gain was so fast people kept not recognizing me. I remember attending regular meetings and no one knew me from one meeting time to the next. It was like being a stranger who needed to be introduced as a new person each time.*
>
> *So, that summer in Coronado was a rude awakening — beginning to really get acquainted with and to assimilate the real me, the new me. I decided not to rent a car, but to get an old beater of a bicycle and use it as my only means of transportation, aside from using buses, also a new experience for me. I rode the bike, and then ran on the beach for exercise. It was a completely glorious summer of being responsible only for me — for simply staying sober, losing weight and taking care of me. I worried not at all about my finances while there, simply concentrated on my health. It felt totally decadent and even selfish. Yet, I knew it was time to be selfish in a healthy manner.*
>
> *While I was running on the street one day, a guy whistled at me. I was so startled when he whistled, I nearly ran into a parked car. I*

thought to myself "What is wrong with these California guys? They're nuts!"

There were lots of young Navy men there. One day I was luxuriating in the apartment complex Jacuzzi when a guy started flirting outrageously with me. Again, I found myself wondering what was wrong with these weird California men. I ran up to my room in a sort of panic, and looked in the mirror. Suddenly, like a ton of bricks, the thought hit me: "Wow — I am not seeing what the rest of the world is seeing. I am still seeing fat!" And boy, was I still seeing fat. It took a long time to get my brain and body in the same space and time. There is still a small, lingering fat person-image inside my brain. Maybe she will always be there?

Later that summer of 1980, I returned to Denver. My husband and I immediately went to a birthday party in a glitzy, gorgeous home in the foothills belonging to one of my contract employees. Her husband didn't recognize me. He came to greet us at the door, said hello to my spouse and then started to shake my hand and introduce himself. Suddenly he shouted, "Oh, my God! Lin, it's you!" He lifted me up off the floor in a huge bear hug, and with gusto danced me around like a big rag doll — shouting to everyone "Look at this! Look at this! It's Lin!" I felt like a million dollars.

For me, asking for help was necessary in all my problem areas. I asked for help when I went to the doctor, then was admitted to the hospital in 1980. I was essentially asking for help for the blood pressure, other physical problems, addictions and weight control.

Although my financial problems were looming on the horizon, they were not clear to me at that time. I did not ask for help on financial matters until quite some time later.

Initially it really doesn't matter who you ask for help. You can ask:

- God, or whatever you believe is a Power higher than you.
- Your best friend.
- Your teacher.
- Your family, spouse, kids.
- A counselor.
- A minister or spiritual guide.
- A group (self-help or otherwise).
- Professional advisors: attorney, CPA, broker.
- Even an enemy.

It's the reaching out that initiates movement and creates commitment to the process. So, do it. Ask for help. Go to the library. Go to a minister, counselor, psychiatrist, doctor, friend, support group, organization, your lover, mother, father, spouse. The important thing is to start.

Are you willing to reach out and to humble yourself to ask for help?

Most of us don't know how to ask for help. We have the idea we shouldn't have to ask, that either others will see our pain or problems and offer to help . . . or offer a solution . . . or rescue us . . . or whatever it is you were brought up to believe. Or we believe we are supposed to have all the answers, know how to handle everything. Or we just are not willing to appear unknowing or vulnerable. That is one of my favorites. I am a small woman who succeeded fairly well in the world of "men in business." Not true, but that's how I saw it. So, if I admitted that I didn't know something — or that I needed help — or didn't know where to get answers or what to do next — someone might take advantage of me, hurt me, get to me. And we couldn't have that now, could we?

One of my recent big lessons about asking for help came in early 1996. I had been hiking a lot. My knee began to hurt seriously when I came down a steep trail. I finally decided to go to a doctor and ended up with a well-known orthopedist. He was "95% sure" that I needed an arthroscopy due to a problem with a meniscus, very likely from horseback riding, falls, and a history of tumbling team falls in high school. This simple procedure should be able to correct the problem and I could get on with hiking and all the rest of the activities that I love.

Talk about interesting choices. I previously had chosen a cheap insurance when I no longer had corporate coverage. I ended up in a mobile, day-surgery setting; they had no laser, which, as it turned out, could have helped greatly. Instead of a repairable meniscus problem, the doctor found severe arthritis. Without a laser to create some bleeding and tissue damage so that new, healthier tissue would form, basically nothing could be done. The doctor told me knee replacement would be my only option and that I should do all the activities I most loved, as much as I could, as soon as I could. I was devastated.

I had been meeting a group of mutually-supportive women once a week. Before the surgery I told them what was happening. I was very upset when no one called to check on me and ask how I was doing. The next week, when my friend Mo called to see if I was attending the group, I said "No. I was pretty disgusted that no one cared enough to call."

I will not soon forget Mo's reply: "Gee, Lin, let's think about that. What you did was show up smiling as usual, acting as though everything was handled and under control. You seemed absolutely OK with it all."

"Everything is not all right," I said. "I needed your support! How am I supposed to get it?!"

My loving friend answered, "Perhaps you could ask for support when you need it!"

Perhaps.

When I was finally faced with the reality that my business had indeed been embezzled and that bankruptcy was imminent if I didn't make yet another considerably significant change, I was faced with asking for help again. In reality, my financial turnaround has been nearly as pivotal as all the other changes in my experience.

Talk about more interesting choices! I had not been reading my own financial statements regularly; I was not even signing the corporate checks or paychecks myself. The only time I had information about the corporation's financial status was when my bookkeeper/accountant prepared a financial statement for me to take to the bank to sign personally for a loan.

I was dealing with some pretty sizeable reimbursement problems, both in the rehab agency and the home health agency. I had a second lien on my home and didn't know where to turn. An attorney I met with said, "Bankruptcy is not the answer to your problems. Here is the reality: You will not be keeping that nice diamond on your finger. You will not be driving that lovely sports car. You will not be living in that nice house on the hill. My advice is: Stop spending like there is no tomorrow. Go home and cut up your credit cards. Start saving. Live differently and take responsibility for your finances."

Good advice. Thank you, John.

My husband was an over-spender, too. That also came to an end. We were both accustomed to large salaries and huge benefits. We had no savings and had barely started an IRA for retirement. We were accustomed to spending it all.

Another significant consultant also helped me turn my finances around. This CPA asked me, "How do you spend all you make?"

I didn't even understand the question! "What do you mean?" I asked. "We buy toys, cars, houses, eat out a lot, travel a lot, play a lot."

I don't understand what happened in my brain. I know my parents were savers, so I must have grown up around that kind of thinking. I know they were appalled by the way my husband and I blew all our money.

I stopped doing two things: over-spending and spending money I didn't have. I stopped being married to a man who did the same. I began taking responsibility for my own financial future, not waiting for someone else to fix it. I began investing in my own retirement, even when I thought I couldn't afford it.

The CPA had a huge impact on my life. Dave taught me to read the Wall Street Journal. He taught me to protect my business from embezzlement. He led me into knowing that having money is not evil. He walked me through deal-making and selling my business. Thank you, Dave.

As you can see, in the financial arena, asking for help meant consulting extensively with a CPA and an attorney, then changing nearly all of my concepts and beliefs about money and abundance. It meant putting away credit cards and not spending money we didn't have. It was the beginning of the eventual decision to sell my practice, but before that could happen, many things had to take place to give sufficient value to the corporation — so someone would be willing to pay a good price for it.

I must admit that learning to spend differently, both personally and professionally, was as challenging a new behavior as all the other health and addiction "new behaviors" and choices. My financial turnaround was largely a function of improved management: the hiring of excellent consultants followed by a willingness to do what they suggested, letting problem people, contracts, and concepts go, and then enlisting the help of all my wonderful employees. If I had been blessed with spectacular skills in management, they were along the line of hiring the most amazing people. The employees were astounding! If I was willing to contribute 100%, they seemed willing to participate at 110%.

But, even more challenging was all there was to learn after the sale of my business. Oh, my. I didn't know a stock from a bond from a future or an option. I didn't know a money manager from a broker. I returned to Denver after closing the sale of my business with big checks in hand and in a complete panic about how to start learning about investing. I was elated, yet scared and overwhelmed.

I sold the company on October 1, 1987, and had no idea where to start — even where to put the money while I learned enough to start making investment decisions. I got lucky in that I had a (different) stock broker who gave me a dose of reality and humility. "Oh, Lin," she said, "it is no big deal. I have clients who keep that much money liquid! Since you don't know what you want to do we will put the cash in double tax exempt government bonds."

It couldn't have been a better decision, for 20 days later the market bombed. I could have lost pretty much everything (and this was prior to paying taxes on the business sales proceeds.) As it was, I lost over $100,000 just in the price drop of the stock in the corporation that acquired mine. It was an interesting time to start learning how to ask for help and get responsible about money!

Then I hired my first money manager. She told me something very important about investing: "Lin, if you can just remember two things about investing and the stock market, it will serve you well. Two emotions govern the market: fear and greed." I have kept that information in front of me for all my future capital decisions. It has served me well.

In a nutshell: what asking for financial help meant in the business turnaround was finding, interviewing, then hiring the best possible accountants, attorneys, consultants and having an effective board of directors for the corporation. It meant ask, learn, then ask and learn some more.

After the business sale, it meant add to those consultants a patient and good-communicating money manager and stock broker/investment counselor. In my opinion, a good broker does not work for a company who pushes certain products because of their high commissions, but who knows my whole monetary picture and helps me make decisions based on long-term goals.

I continue to ask for lots of help from these important consultants in my life, and to accept responsibility for my fiscal condition. What that now means to me is an awareness that:

- Money is only money, and although I deserve to be comfortable and as secure as possible, security is a spiritual quality and not a matter of having a certain number of dollars (it can all be gone in a minute and does not connote quality of life).

- Money in and of itself is not evil, in fact can be used for a lot of good; the love and idolization of money and stuff is dangerous and not an ideal for me.

- I could not wait for someone else to fix my money problems years ago, and I cannot expect anyone else to take charge of my fiscal responsibilities now.

- I personally have to maintain on-going watchfulness and awareness on a regular and disciplined basis: i.e., meet with my consultants regularly and read all account statements as they arrive to look for patterns or problem areas.

- I can't blame anyone else for past or present fiscal results.
- I have to ask questions, continue to learn and read.
- I must pay attention to what is going on in the business and financial world, while not obsessing about all the ups and downs which are inevitable.
- I must also understand that all investments have risk (life is risky!).
- I must also lose my fear of and/or guilt about wealth or a lack thereof.

It is interesting to observe that we human beings will tell each other all about our sex lives, sexual preferences, addictions, past abuses, family stuff, bodies, diseases, travels, kids, marriages, and many more personal experiences, yet seldom are we comfortable talking directly and clearly about money. I don't know if that comes from messages such as "Don't ever ask how much he makes. Don't ask how much they are worth. Never ask what something costs. Money is personal."

I made a decision to share more information about the miracle of my own financial reverses in this book because I have come to understand that more people have these problems than I knew. A lot of people seem to be seeking attitude changes and practical suggestions for their financial problems.

Since my first book came out, I have realized from people telling me their stories how many people have huge credit card debt and truly do live from paycheck to paycheck. This seems to apply to people who have very high paying jobs as well as those who own their own businesses and/or have lower paying jobs. There seems to be a need, especially among many

Americans who earn a lot, to display a lavish lifestyle. We are a nation of high-consumption and high-debt lifestyles. We love to display our wealth.

I've enjoyed reading a most interesting book entitled "The Millionaire Next Door," by Thomas Stanley and William Danko (Longstreet Press, 1998, Marietta, Georgia). One of the main points is that we all probably know millionaires who do not display a lifestyle which would make us think they are. They do not drive a new Lexus, their house is paid for, they do not wear a $15,000 Rolex, nor do they wear custom-made expensive suits.

The typical profile of the millionaire next door is small business owner, one or two generations emigrated from a much more conservative (and frugal) country and culture, who drinks beer not champagne and dresses more like his or her employees than like a VIP. Another key characteristic is s/he is debt-free, or nearly so.

If you are utilizing a few of the ideas in this book to choose different financial results for yourself, I would truly suggest you add "The Millionaire Next Door" to your reading list. My book and these 7 Keys will help you make a mental and emotional break-through, or commitment to create different results, and other materials can help you learn exactly what to do. None of us has to be poor in spirit or in financial matters. Not in the United States of America.

Today, asking for help means to me: having people in my life who hold me accountable and keep me on track; staying involved with my friends instead of wandering off on my own, while learning all the new things required to write, publish and market another book — at the same time advancing a professional speaking career. It means hiring help for all the things I can't do.

Where am I now financially? I am in a solid-enough monetary position to work part-time, learn new skills, write a book, and record tapes. Writing a book and hiring editor, designer, illustrator, publicist, etc., costs a lot of money and I can loan myself the money. That is pretty amazing, isn't it?

Accept Responsibility

The second half of this third Key is "accept responsibility." It means that we must accept responsibility for all our choices. An interesting phenomenon occurs in recovery from addictions. Many addicts and alcoholics come from very religious backgrounds and attempt to address their alcoholism, addictions, and issues by returning to the church or religion of their childhood. Then they can't figure out why — if God or a Higher Power is required for recovery — the church didn't work?

In my opinion and by my long-term observation, as wonderful as the grace of God is, unless and until recovering persons take responsibility for the messes they have made of their lives, jobs, marriages, finances, health, past and present, all the grace in the universe will not solve their problems nor move them into recovery. They must do the clean-up and take action or the grace is not effective.

If you accept that no matter what it is that you want to change, you did something to cause it by putting yourself in that position — knowingly or unknowingly, consciously or unconsciously — and you realize that you must do all it takes to create a different result, then you are beginning to accept personal responsibility for your life and choices. So how do you follow through?

Accepting responsibility means doing all it takes to create a different result.

When I weighed 200 pounds and wanted to lose 70, I wanted to just think differently or pray myself thin. You know what? No matter how much I prayed, God never did come down and push me away from the table or run me around the block or lift the weights for me! I could not just diet . . . or just pray . . . just exercise . . . or just think differently . . . or do differently for a short period of time. That's why diet guru Richard Simmons calls it a "live-it" not a diet. A life change means doing all it takes for as long as it takes to create a different result. Most cases of desired change mean for the rest of our lives!

I was privileged to participate with my dear mother in her recovery from cancer. There was a point in her disease when she made a conscious decision to do all it would take to recover. She would not give up. When looking out over the canyon in the backyard, near the beautiful San Isabel National Forest in southern Colorado, she decided that she had the love of her family and a life worth living and she was not about to give up until she was ready. She decided then to do all it would take for the best possibility of recovery.

That meant having surgery to remove the diseased part of her body, then a radiation implant, which produced difficult side effects such as stomach and intestinal problems. Her recovery to normalcy has been long and slow. She must be constantly vigilant and take the best care of herself she can. She has had to adopt new behaviors. I asked her to try something else new to her — mental imaging, to mentally visualize the "good" white cells gobbling up the "bad" cancer cells. Many fervent prayers were said on her behalf, also. And we were blessed, the miracle happened.

Was, is it all worth it? Yes. At the times when she suffers the side effects of the radiation, I know she wonders whether it is worth it. However, being the person she is, I don't believe she would have done differently.

My Mom recently brought her 94-year-old mother into her own marriage of 53 years, to live with them. My parents added a room to their home to accommodate Grandma during her last years. My Mom is finding strength she — and we — didn't know she had. She asked for help and now continues to accept responsibility for her own recovery and ongoing health.

My father has had his recovery issues as well. He was seriously burned when he was preparing to go four-wheeling with Mom and friends. The jeep wouldn't start. Mom cranked the starter while Dad threw gasoline on the carburetor. The gasoline exploded, and Dad tossed the can into the air. Gasoline came down all over him, burning 20-25% of his upper body with second and third degree burns. He was wearing a polyester jumpsuit which melted to him. He rolled on the ground to put out the fire.

Most definitely, my dad did not knowingly cause this accident. No one else did it to him, either. Blame is not the issue. The accident seems to have been the result of unconscious actions or choices without proper caution and forethought to possible consequences.

Dad made sound choices with the event of the accident. He rolled on the ground; went to the hospital; took the medicine, the physical therapy, whirlpools; and got the necessary skin grafts. Going to visit my dad and seeing him in terrible pain is an experience I never want again. Burns are horrible! I will never forget the smell of his burned flesh. My mom will never forget the sight of him on fire.

My dad certainly had to ask for help and accept responsibility for his actions. Today he is a very active 76-year-old man. He still tills his gardens, wrestles calves, and throws hay bales. He goes fishing in Alaska.

I learned that life without crutches can be difficult. In the old days I dealt with good and bad stuff by escaping the fear or pain; by abusing food, alcohol and pills; by spending a lot and living the highest possible lifestyle. Now, I find that one of the hardest things about major change, or giving up a lot of old unhealthy "crutches" is learning to deal with life head on. Do you know what I mean?

> *When Mom was diagnosed with cancer, I went through the denial, anger and all that it took to be in the best possible mental space for her — without the crutches. It was hard. It was also one of the most frightening things I can remember. I can't even imagine what it was like for her, or my dad. What I won't ever forget, though, is my heart leaping into my throat as we walked down the hospital hall and confronted the orange-gold and black sign on the*

wall which said "RADIATION." I thought, "Oh dear God. My mother really has cancer. She is here to have that stuff put into her body!"

Dad wanted me to stay with him at their lovely mountain home, in Rye, Colorado. After spending the night, Dad wanted to go for an early morning walk in the canyon together. It was rare and delightful to have Dad all to myself, so I happily said "Of course!" It was quiet and sunny, with fresh mountain air, abundant wildlife and birdsong.

Afterward we went back to the hospital to see Mom. She had just come out of surgery and was lying alone on a pram, eyes closed, in the cold and very dreary gray hospital hall. She was as gray as the walls, and her cheeks had two very plain tear-tracks down them. She had not yet received her pain medication. She was so still and unresponsive, I thought for sure she was dead. Apparently, Dad did too. He let out a wailing sob and crumpled to the floor, holding onto the side of her pram.

This little girl and only daughter had seldom seen her father cry! My heart shattered into a million pieces of pain for him . . . and for her . . . and for me . . . and for the helplessness and hopelessness of it all. I was overwhelmed with a sudden comprehension of the strength of love that bound these two people, my parents, after more then 40 years of marriage. I couldn't imagine one without the other. Thankfully, I didn't have to, for she was as OK as could be expected under the circumstances.

In many ways, that hospital did very badly by us. Whole wings of the hospital were closed down and many on the staff didn't seem to be involved in nurturing a patient beyond the basics. When Mom went to surgery to have radiation implanted, no one told us what to expect. Nobody told her anything.

I stood frozen in shock when she was returned to her room and the entire room, ceiling, walls, and floor were lined with newspaper to absorb the radiation which had been implanted in her. It was worse than grim. We couldn't touch her. We couldn't hug her. We had to stand behind a lead shield to talk to her and protect us from her radiation! Her Bible and all her precious reading materials were gone. Her clothes were gone. Everything had been cleared out. She was catheterized and had to remain on her back in bed for several days.

I don't know if she was too sick to be angry but I was furious. How dare they treat her that way and not even prepare her? I went out to purchase helium-filled balloons so they would float up to the ceiling so she would have something to look at. And I wrapped a large box in colorful paper containing 14 individually wrapped and decorated gifts for her to have one to look forward to each day.

The point is that when we ask for help, accept responsibility for the tough stuff, and enough love, faith, and healing are present — when the process of change and its results are at their best — we very human beings can handle just about anything. And we can handle it without "crutches." We simply face it and go through it minute by minute, day by day, sometimes month by month. We pray. We ask for help and accept responsibility — again and again. We feel the pain and fear and acknowledge it.

I am so grateful to have gone through all that with my parents while I was sober, clean and doing no destructive or bingeing behavior. I did not have to climb back into a bottle of alcohol, or box of chocolates, or a bottle of Valium to deal with real life and death issues. It seemed like a miracle but, in reality, was simply asking for help and accepting responsibility.

How are you doing? What do you need help with? Better communication with your children, spouse, family? Ending of a relationship? Anger, resentment, fear? Abuse, drugs, alcohol? A business venture, an old job, a new job? Friends, lovers, money? The past, present, future?

What do you need to accept responsibility for? Your marriage? Your money? Your past? I don't know the answer. But you do. You can do all it takes to create a different result. You can create positive change. I know that if I can, you can.

Asking for help and taking responsibility are not just one-time events. You can't just take responsibility for your marriage . . . or your anger . . . or your weight solely for today. While, it is true that today is the only day you can live and change, taking responsibility means changing every single day. For good. Forever. That attitude and behavior brings the lasting successful result.

The good news is: One day at a time is all you can do and anybody can change one habit for one day. All those single days add up to a changed habit. I have heard that to change a habit we need to change how we do something seven times. I have no empirical or scientific evidence to substantiate that, but if we drive to work a different route seven trips in a row, we are well on our way to creating a new habit of driving to work. Other experts have said it takes 21 days or 28 days to establish a new habit. No matter. What else were you planning to do with the next 28 days?

I do know I can't lose a pound yesterday. I can't lose a pound tomorrow. But I can lose a pound today. I can not drug or drink today. I can spend and invest responsibly today. I can ask for help today. I can accept responsibility today. So can you.

How exactly do we accept responsibility for our choices? We clean up our pasts after acknowledging that we made choices that put us where we are today. Then we do all we can one day at a time to change the results. When we want to reduce our weight, we make a lifestyle change forever — one day at a time. To change being habitually late, we accept the consequences of our past behavior, learn new behaviors, do all it takes to change and live differently each day.

Webster's Dictionary says responsibility is being reliable, trustworthy, stable. Sometimes responsibility is merely the "ability to respond."

In Colorado we periodically have major hail storms. I have experienced two such destructive storms in my years as a homeowner. I have had to replace the shake shingles of two homes, re-paint both homes and make other numerous repairs due to the severity of these summer disasters.

Perhaps you have had the same experience. If your responsibility is to clean up after a hail storm, even though you'd rather not, if you choose to live in an area where hail storms happen often, responsibility is the ability to respond after a hail storm. This applies in many instances when we truly want to say "I am not responsible for this!"

Responsibility:
Ability to respond.
Positively.

Ask for help and accept responsibility for your choices:

- Asking for help is essential to the change process.
- So is accepting responsibility for your choices.
- If you are not willing to ask for help, you will stay in your same patterns of behavior.
- There is help available for every area you may want to change.
- Accepting responsibility means doing *all* it takes to create new or different results — a day at a time.

Any system which takes responsibility away from people, dehumanizes them.

— Dr. Robert Anthony

Your Turn

1. Who and in what area(s) of my life do I need to ask for help?

2. In which areas of my life am I now willing to accept responsibility for undesirable results from past choices? *(Be honest, no one else needs to see this.)*

3. Am I willing to accept responsibility for new or different results both now and in the future?

I believe that every right implies a responsibility; every opportunity, an obligation; every possession, a duty.

— John D. Rockefeller

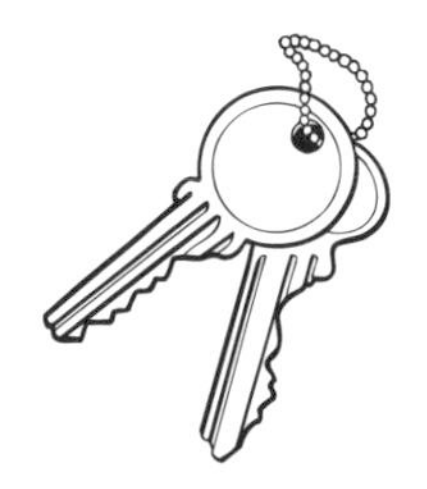

Key # 4:

Never Quit!

The path of least resistance is simply giving up. The world and society often don't want us to succeed. Have you heard a lot more about what you **can't** do than what you **can** do?

The world's greatest feats have been accomplished by very persistent people as noted in "Chicken Soup for the Soul" by Mark V. Hansen and Jack Canfield:

- Babe Ruth, considered by many to be one of the greatest athletes of all time, is famous for setting the home run record. He also struck out 1330 times.
- Eighteen publishers turned down Richard Bach's 10,000 word story about a "soaring" seagull, Jonathan Livingston Seagull. Macmillan finally published it in 1970. By 1975, it had sold over seven million copies in the U.S. alone.

- Henry Ford went broke five times before he finally succeeded.
- Winston Churchill failed sixth grade. When he was 62 he became the prime minister of England after a lifetime of defeats. He made his greatest contributions as a "senior citizen."

Don't quit
Keep going!

I desperately wanted dieting to be a one-time event. But it isn't! I have surrendered to the fact that watching my diet and exercising is forever — as are all the other improvements in my life. If I think, "I can never drink again . . . never eat what I want again . . . never be in love again," I am overwhelmed and incredibly discouraged. The only successful way to do any change is:

- Make a decision.
- Practice, practice, practice.
- Apply all the other things you've read so far and what is yet to come in this book.
- Do each new behavior and way of thinking one day at a time!

Forever is too long for our minds to grasp. We can handle one day at a time.

> *Just as I was beginning to understand and utilize this concept, I found myself running past a bakery in downtown Coronado almost every day. Fresh-made brownies beckoned to me from the front window. Oh boy, do I love chocolate brownies! And I loved them even*

more during that summer of 1980. They were thick, moist, chewy, deep, dark chocolate, covered in delicious, abundant, rich fudge icing. Some even had nuts on them. Cravings set in. I thought I would die without a brownie. The more I thought about them, the more I had to have them. Not just one, of course, several . . . If I just had one of anything, at that time, my thinking would start to sound something like this: "Oh well, I have already broken my diet. Might as well just forget it for today and eat anything I want."

One day the thought popped into my mind: "They tell me just not to drink ***today.*** *Not to worry about yesterday or tomorrow. Maybe that will work for brownies, too. The bakers seem to make those brownies every day. They have had that recipe for years and been making these same brownies for years. They will probably make them tomorrow, and the next day, and the next. I guess I will just choose not to have brownies today. Maybe tomorrow, but not today." Then, of course, one tomorrow every two weeks or so, would become a today, and I rewarded myself with a brownie.*

Deprivation is such a huge psychological aspect of "giving up" or learning major changes like not drinking, not drugging, stopping over-spending, or changing eating habits in a big way. If you allow the feeling of deprivation it will lead to self-pity and that is truly dangerous. If we don't find other body-and-soul, completely satisfying substitutes for our cravings, we emotionally shrivel up and die on the vine. I found a little store with stems-on, huge, red, juicy strawberries dipped in chocolate. They were not nearly as big a cheat as a brownie, yet still made me feel that I had eaten something very special and rewarding. Feelings of deprivation and self-pity were not necessary. I still have to do some of those same things today.

A few of my food compulsions still show up today. They are greatest when I am on the road — especially when I travel to speak or consult. If the plane is late, or the weather is bad, or the speaking/room set-up is all wrong, or the people are a bit challenging, or I forgot some paperwork, or my audio tapes and books didn't show up with me and my other luggage . . . I have discovered I still have the belief in my little brain that food is wired up with reward for effort or stress. I don't know why. I don't understand it. I never remember my parents using food as a reward or prize or punishment. Where does that come from? Perhaps food is simply comforting when it goes beyond our actual needs.

I have accepted that I probably always will have those times when chocolate, or sugar, or heavily buttered, salted popcorn at the movie is an absolute necessity. And I have learned it is OK. My body just cannot expect it all day, every day.

When I arrived in Ohio one night before a seminar I was to lead, I found three huge, freshly baked cookies in my room with a tall glass of milk. It was a very unique and lovely "welcome" room service item. I ate them, of course, while skipping dinner to compensate.

After two very long, challenging days and my first-ever keynote address, I was exhausted. I was also exhilarated, excited, thrilled and amazed to see people walking around for the rest of the time I was there, carrying my book, and especially, reading it while working out in the exercise room.

But the seminar room was all wrong the second day and the woman who had hired me, while using her considerable persuasive skills to negotiate my fee downward, now suddenly was not very accommodating. Twice as many people showed up as planned. I didn't have enough personality profiles — and they cannot be duplicated. It was challenging to say the least.

Intensely weary afterward, I began packing up boxes, stuffing papers into my briefcase, keeping track of checks, charge slips and cash. My hostess arrived with a lovely thank you gift. It was a cookie canister filled with Ohio-shaped solid chocolate candies, yogurt and chocolate covered pretzels, and "Buckeyes." Buckeyes are the pod of an indigenous Ohio tree and the nickname for Ohioans. These candies were amazingly decadent, rich solid creamy butter/peanut butter mounds, surrounded by a soft shell of chocolate — yes, chocolate. Each was wrapped individually, and they were on the top of all the rest — precious as pure gold. I am pretty sure each one of those luscious tidbits contained at least 600 calories and 50 fat grams.

They were perfect rewards for my stress level and tired body and brain. Did I eat them? You betcha. In fact, I ate quite a few. I brought the rest home and gave some to the neighbors who picked up my mail in my absence. (See, I think it is a reward for them, too.) My still-skewed thinking goes along the lines of "Waste not, want not!" "It was so thoughtful, I can't just throw them out!" "How much weight could I gain in only one day if I ate them almost all at once?"

Oh, come on now, don't laugh at me. You've had thoughts like that yourself!

Never quit means to keep going, get rid of your negative thoughts and beliefs. Your family or teachers or someone else in authority may have taught you to not get your hopes up, so you wouldn't be disappointed — or some such thing. Our culture reinforces the negative and minimizes the positive. It is up to you to maximize the positive.

For evidence of that, all you have to do is turn on the news. Some newscasts think that one small piece of good news (e.g., five minutes out of two hours) is enough. When I catch myself believing that the world really is destroying itself, I stop listening to the news. If we go to war or the stock market crashes and I go broke, I figure someone will let me know.

Thinking positively is a very necessary, big part of any changes we wish to make in our lives. But it must be accompanied by positive action. The action is essential even though it involves risk and major effort. Then, we must seek out positive people — and, happily, there are more and more every day. They understand "Change your thinking, change your life." I choose to spend my time with positive thinkers and action types. They understand positive acts and random acts of kindness. They truly produce immense and significant changes on this planet. And you and I can, too!

To keep going, to inspire you to never quit is to surround yourself with inspirational books and movies. Find material that inspires you.

When I need a boost to get positive or to get in touch with myself I go for a hike, preferably in the mountains. When I had to cut back on my high country hiking, I bought an old four wheel drive GMC (Jimmy). I call him "Sir James" and he has good days and bad days, so I am very kind to him and treat him with the utmost respect so he will be good to me.

One summer day I had finished a two-day consulting session with clients in Keystone, Colorado. "James" and I headed east out of

Keystone to a little town called Montezuma. I especially love to do this during the week, when fewer people are on the roads and trails. I turned south up a very rough and rocky trail to Saints John, a big defunct silver mining area, named for Saint John the Baptist and Saint John the Evangelist. The trail gets very steep, narrow and exciting. It also gets very windy higher up on the mountain above Saints John.

I was delighted when I found a remote trail, even further off the beaten track where no one but one or two horses and perhaps one other hiker had been all season. The spring runoff offered the clear fresh sound of a rushing mountain stream. There were millions of wild flowers, pure, clear cobalt Colorado sky, and not another soul on the trail. Now that is heaven! It reminds me that anything is possible. I just have to believe and keep going.

Another excellent way to bolster your positive energy is to read great books. I recently read an autobiography about Todd Huston, "More Than Mountains: The Todd Huston Story." I hope to meet this awesome man some day. He is on my list of 101 goals!

At the age of 14, Todd was boating when his legs got caught in the boat propeller. Ongoing medical problems forced him to choose amputation at the age of 21. It would have been simpler for him — and very acceptable to society — to spend the rest of his life in a wheelchair. Instead, he was obsessed with the desire to overcome mountains, literally and figuratively. He challenged a climbing record held by an able-bodied man. He sought to climb the highest peak in each of the 50 United States in one hundred days or less!

He climbed through the pain of a misfit prosthesis, friction irritation, bleeding, and skin problems. His triumph was climbing to the top of Mt. McKinley in Alaska! I have hiked 12 times up to 14,000 feet; easy walk-up "Fourteeners." Whenever I feel sorry for myself because at my age my little hiking career is probably coming to a close because of severe arthritis in my knees, I think of Todd Huston. He did it! I can do it, too. So, I keep hiking.

It helps to surround ourselves with inspiration on every level. As a lover of the outdoors, hiking, and climbing, I recommend the movie, "K-2," about conquering a 28,000-foot-high mountain in the Himalayas. I have probably viewed this movie more than five times. It always thrills, scares, and inspires me with its powerful message of persistence, wanting something enough to die for it, about people working together to overcome obstacles, and finally, about surviving against all odds.

There is real power in knowing that if others can, you can!

A great spiritual principle is "What I focus on, expands." If you focus on everything you cannot do, that is all you can see. You just see more and more of what you absolutely cannot do. Self-pity sets in.

If you focus on everything you can do, that is what you see. You then get to live in gratitude and abundance. It is your choice.

This concept keeps showing up in my life. For example, I was riding my bike recently on a concrete path about eight feet wide. I saw a bug ahead on the path, off to one side. I definitely did not want to hit and squash it. Of course the mere act of noticing it and meaning to miss it drew my energy — and front tire — right to it.

"How could that be," I wondered, "when I meant to miss it?" It demonstrated perfectly the principle of "What I look toward, I go toward." I have to remember that principle also applies to all the good, positive changes I want to make, too.

You are absolutely where you are supposed to be! You have enough of everything — right now! Tomorrow is a new day. Tomorrow is full of creative solutions — and so are you.

That also applies to the people with whom you surround yourself. I expected my friends and family to say, "What? You can't write a book. Don't be silly." Not one of them, even my CPAs and attorneys (you know, those people we actually pay to keep us cautious?) told me I couldn't. Every person said, "Go for it. You can do it." Wow! I have made good choices in my friends.

Never Quit:

- Never quit means you must keep on keeping on until the results are altered for good.
- It means keeping on one minute, hour, day at a time.
- Thinking positively is all-important.
- Surrounding ourselves with positive, uplifting, encouraging people and material helps us not quit or give up.
- What I focus on expands, so I must focus on "I can!"

Whatever you want, wants you.

— Dr. Robert Anthony

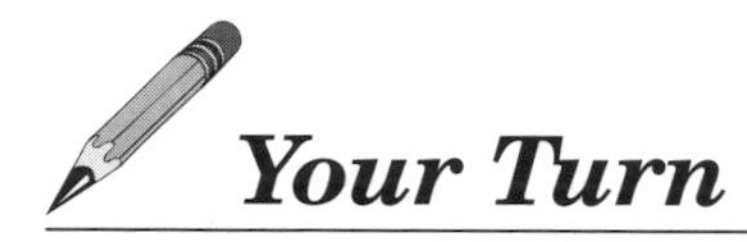

Your Turn

1. Where am I most tempted to quit, to give up?

2. What's the first step I can take to quit quitting?

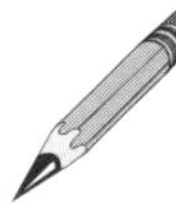

Your Turn

3. Make a contract with yourself, now. Put your commitment into writing. Thoughts are powerful, action creates results.

I, ______________________________ ,
am committed to

____.

Each time I am tempted to give up, I will

____.

I do this because I am worthy of a happy, healthy, prosperous and fulfilled life.

____________________ ____________________

Date Signature

All things must change
To something new, to
Something strange.

— Longfellow

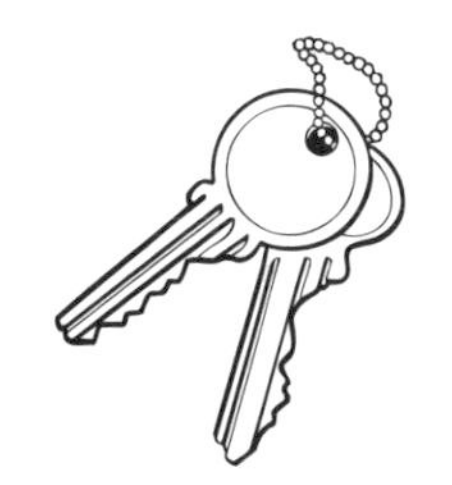

Key # 5:

Grab On to the New, Let Go of the Old

For change to be real and lasting we must make conscious decisions, commitments to let go of old ways of thinking, doing, being, living. Since we cannot hold both the old and the new at the same time, we absolutely must let go of the old in order to create mental, emotional, spiritual or physical space for new habits, ideas, patterns, and possibilities. Letting go must be completely without reservation.

I have frequently heard, “Anything I finally let go of still has claw marks all over it!” Most of us have a difficult time “letting go.” We like our lives familiar and comfortable. We don’t want changes we don’t understand or know how to do well, or that upset our routines. When I was in the throes of my alcohol addiction, I didn’t want to try anything I was not already good at. I didn’t want to be embarrassed. I didn’t want to look bad. My sense of humor was stifled! I mean, I was important. I was the Boss. I couldn't laugh at myself.

How I've changed! Today, I don't care who laughs at me. And they do. I am willing to try anything new which excites me, enhances my life, doesn't hurt anyone else and doesn't hurt me. My sense of humor and daring have led me to do some foolhardy things. However, I have learned to let go of the old and grab onto the new. Fun and laughter are a big part of my life today.

Letting go of old ideas, my old way of life, old loves, and my physical therapy practice were very hard releases. I was "married" to my business twice as long as either spouse. The business was my life and my identity. Sometimes I still miss the socialization of the office setting and being needed on a daily basis.

It was so strange the first Christmas without my business not to be part of deciding what we would do differently than the 16 Christmas celebrations before. Would we be able to pay cash bonuses to employees? Should we do a sleigh ride? Dinner party? Home party? Have gifts? Draw names? I felt totally lost without the big celebration. I had a hard time letting go of the status and connection. I also had a hard time letting go of the income, the steady predictable paycheck. That showed me how much my identity was connected to how much money I made. Even my self-esteem was determined by my paycheck.

Finally I was able to let go of the need to be a boss — the authority and center of my little universe. I moved into a much more solitary situation — a home office.

What helps you make a decision and transition into something new?

- Get clear that letting go is important and indeed necessary.
- Ask for help.
- Clear your mental and emotional space for something new.
- Look for something to replace your old way of living, being, doing.

Old things you might have to let go of:

- Old ideas, such as: “That’s just the way it is . . . That’s the way it has always been . . . Because I said so.”
- Excuses for being the way you are: “That just the way I am! My grandmother was that way . . . My father is that way . . .”
- Old loves. It seems to take at least a year to heal and really let go.
- Identity based on expense accounts, position, title.
- Job identities. You are more than just a doctor, dentist, secretary, stockbroker, lawyer, business owner, parent, homemaker.
- Identity based on someone else in your life: wife, husband, mother, father.
- Money, things, and their connection to who you are.
- Who everyone else thinks you are or ought to be.
- Past family experiences: for example, you are this way because you were victimized, abused, etc.

Many of us let go by extending a hand in front of us, palm up with open fingers, stating “I am willing to let go.” This reserves an “out” for us. We can close our fingers and take back our old ideas and behaviors whenever we get too uncomfortable.

To let go for good, extend your hand in front of you palm down. Open your fingers and release downward. Gravity takes over and the ideas, thoughts, and behaviors are gone beyond your ability to take them back. This is “Letting go and Letting God.”

No matter what your spiritual belief, to change your personal or business life, it helps to access a Higher Power — whatever that is for you. Frequently there comes a time when you personally have done all you can to improve yourself and your situation and you have to let go again! It is my experience that the grace of God helps in this process. "Be patient," I say to myself — and my friends — "God isn't finished with me yet!"

Selfishness was and still is my very human trait. Personal awareness and growth has taken a lot of effort. It helped me immensely to get busy helping others. During the times of my biggest and most challenging decisions, I often felt sorry for myself. My self-absorption became all consuming. I was all wrapped up in myself. That makes a very small package.

After I sold my therapy company, I was lost, disconnected. No one felt sorry for me. And no one would play the pity game with me. To others I appeared to be suddenly wealthy, but it's all relative! I had three years of payments and interest coming in so I could travel and play. I found that what I focused on, expanded. When I focused on change and loss, I hurt. When I focused on fun and new things, I got to do them.

And I did. I learned to scuba dive, then took a trip to the Seychelles islands 1000 miles east of Nairobi to learn underwater photography. I fell in love with diving! I swam with an 11-foot gray whale shark (the largest fish on the planet), learned to night dive, and did my first wreck dive.

> *My first night dive became a major adventure! On the way to the site a woman shared her first terror-filled night dive story with me. I am sure that didn't help me relax. My dive buddy was also our group leader, my trip roommate, and my photography teacher. She was so confident of my diving skills that once we entered the dark and disorienting sea, she focused on taking her own great photos. The problem was that she ignored me — a relative novice.*
>
> *Because of low-back surgery I cannot wear a typical weight belt diving but have my weights in the pocket of my buoyancy compen-*

sator. In my fear and frustration I inadvertently tripped the cord which released the weights, leaving me no ability to stay underwater. After taking a few very nice night photos of anemone "open" and feeding, and numerous wondrously bright-colored, dark-eyed squirrel fish, I floated to the surface. There I was out in the middle of the Indian Ocean all by myself in the dark and scared to death! I shouted at the boat operators to help. They shouted back, "What are you doing on the surface?!"

"I don't know!" I yelled. "I don't want to be here!"

They were not happy with me for losing those weights. Because of the islands' location so far from the mainland, getting sufficient supplies of heavy dive weights is no small feat!

I also experienced my first near-disaster dive in the Seychelles. A divemaster and another newly-certified diver accompanied me through an eight-foot-diameter tunnel in the granite, on the ocean floor. There was a very strong, difficult surge (current) that jerks you strongly one direction, stops, then throws you the opposite direction.

We caught the surge, strategically passing through the tunnel into a box-canyon-shaped area. A nurse shark was sleeping under some low rocks. The divemaster and I were concerned about the new diver and what her reaction might be to a shark. If she panicked, we were in trouble. Although a nurse shark is virtually harmless, it is still a shark and deserves respect and space.

We started snapping photos while keeping an eye on the possible predator as well as the inexperienced diver. It turned out she didn't

> *even realize what we were seeing was a shark! We managed to spook it and my heart was pounding nearly out of my chest as the shark swam powerfully in a circle, exiting the box-canyon through the tunnel.*
>
> *It was time to follow the big fish out of this cavern. I was so thrilled and nervous that I caught the current too high on the way back through the tunnel. The force of the water threw me up against the rock at the top of the tunnel, which caught my air line and held me there. Fortunately, I had on a wet suit, which I seldom wear, and had the presence of mind to duck my head and pull the camera toward my body. That action saved my head and camera from being smashed against the rock.*
>
> *I waited for the current to reverse direction, which allowed me to unhook from the rock and get through the tunnel safely. When I reached the boat, I realized what a close call it was.*
>
> *The divemaster shook her head. "I can't believe you weren't killed! Look at your tank and wetsuit!"*
>
> *The tank was partially caved-in by crashing against the rock and the wetsuit looked like someone had poured acid on it — small bits had been torn from it but it still protected me from serious cuts and scrapes.*

This powerful experience assured me that my skills were good and my instincts were perfect for self-preservation. I found this experience very significant in letting go of old ideas and lack of confidence to try new things. I also began to see the importance of becoming willing to "grab onto the new," and the necessity of finding joy doing stimulating, fresh activities. I gained a new awareness that Someone-Up-There was watching over me!

More new things: I went into Kenya on a photography safari in four game parks: Masai Mara Game Reserve (a hot air balloon ride there); Lake Nakuru (hundreds of thousands of brilliantly pink flamingoes); Buffalo Springs National Reserve; and Samburu Reserve.

> *I will never forget the medical and immunization requirements for the trip. Boosters, medication, and shots for just about everything: malaria, yellow fever, cholera, tetanus, polio, measles, typhoid, hepatitis A. Prior to leaving Denver for Africa, I got so sick from one of the shots that my throat closed up and I woke in the middle of the night unable to swallow. I ended up in the hospital emergency room wondering if I would make it to Africa.*
>
> *When I went to Emergency I thought I was dying! The doctor asked where I was going.*
>
> *"The Seychelles," I croaked.*
>
> *He launched into a long, flamboyant description of the area, but his information came from the swimsuit issue of "Sports Illustrated." Funny, he remembered a whole lot more about the swimsuits than the Seychelles!*
>
> *Our plane to Nairobi from New York Kennedy Airport developed computer problems, necessitating an un-planned, overnight stop in Frankfurt, Germany. Our tickets had to be changed, so we could bypass Nairobi and fly directly to the Seychelles. Our trip leader had not led a trip of this magnitude before so she was not prepared for the difficulties we experienced.*
>
> *We were standing in an airport waiting for a non-English speaking agent to process our*

plane tickets: she slowly counted them all, "One . . . two . . . three . . ." Then she agonizingly transferred all the tickets to her other hand and counted them all again, "One . . . two . . . three . . ." (each ticket for the entire group).

She did this several more times before I lost patience and asked our leader, "Don't you think you should do something? Or we'll be standing right here while our plane leaves us behind!" We had already lost a day of diving and everyone was restless.

Maureen, our stunning leader, ran up to the counter, leaped up on it to get right in the face of the agent. We were all left staring at her behind draped over the counter! At that sight we all laughed so hard we almost didn't care if we got our tickets any faster or not.

After selling my business, I found many ways to keep busy. I was 41 years old. I'd had my practice for 17 years and employed over 200 people. My time and energy were consumed. Suddenly I had time and energy — to do what? To learn, to grow, to stretch! Africa was just the beginning. I have been blessed to travel quite a bit and 18 days in Africa was way too short for that trip!

Since that time I have been privileged to take a dive trip regularly with two great women friends. We have had amazing adventures in Belize, Bahamas, Cayman Islands, Turks and Caicos. I have also been diving in Saba (Netherlands Antilles), Guanaja, and Cozumel, Mexico. The joy is beyond description!

Nothing of worth exists in a vacuum. Just letting go of the old doesn't work. We must spend some time determining what to do to replace our old ways. New behaviors and thinking become comfortable by repetition. I learned to play piano when I was a child. What was the key to excellence? Practice, practice, practice. Our bodies, muscles, and brains must get accustomed to the new. For me this applies today to diving, traveling, exercising, eating in a healthy manner, writing a book, developing a whole new career.

In life, it feels as though once we reach a comfort level with a new behavior or way of doing/being, things change and once again we are forced to let go of the old. That's just the way life is. Life is always changing, and we are continually forced to grow and accommodate.

In a global economy with the burgeoning Internet and continuous high-tech changes, we must deal with life changing at a faster and faster pace. Do we truly want the world to stop? Do we truly want to stop making progress? To stop changing means death. I mean to keep growing — and flowing — with change. My new ways of doing/being are the best ever. I'm just getting good at it! I know that I will keep at it for at least one more day — today! I can manage letting go and going forward — today!

So can you. Just for one day at a time. Just grow today. What do you need to let go of today? What do you need to start today? Now, do it. You can.

> *I had two significant friends in my life who thought I should be utilizing my speaking talents to make a living. One had been a very high-profile public person on radio, television and in political circles in Colorado. She had helped us market physical therapy when no one ever thought of having to market that. Mary Lynn thought I should take all I knew about Medicare to Washington, D.C. and be a Medicare lobbyist. Lobbyists can make a lot of money and it seemed quite prestigious. So, I spent some time in D.C. and then decided all the lying, game-playing and drinking might not be a wise route for a newly sober alcoholic.*

The other friend had been one of my employees and urged me to take a course in "Public Speaking for the Professional" shortly after my weight loss. They video taped us at the end of the first of two days. I had never seen myself on videotape before. People kept saying I could be a great speaker, that I knew what I was talking about, that I should pursue professional speaking. But, I was horrified when I saw myself on screen!

The teacher noticed that I was acting strangely at the end of the first day. As I was leaving she said, "Lin, you're not coming back, are you?"

"No, Ma'am!" I replied emphatically.

"Don't you think we should talk about it?" she asked gently.

Again, "No, Ma'am!"

She pursued it further and eventually I sat down to discuss my issue with her.

I came to realize that what was so scary was that there was no fat to hide behind. I had a body again and nothing to disguise the fact that I only had two chins and breasts and a face. It felt like such brazen exposure.

With the encouragement and urging of the instructor and my friend, Debbie, I did go back to complete the course. I learned to look at and listen to myself. I learned to even like what I saw. I faced the new me. In order to do that I had to let go of the image of the old me and be willing to deal with all the risks and vulnerability of the new one.

However, some of the letting go of the old image I had of myself was not a single happening or a single awareness. It came in bits and pieces.

As I was re-acquainting myself with me and my loved ones late in the summer of that summer of 1980, my parents and I were in a restaurant. It was the first time in years that I felt free to complete a meal with an ice cream sundae dressed in chocolate syrup, nuts, and topped with whipped cream. What was so astounding about it was that I could now have such a treat without that unbelievably acute awareness of what people were thinking as they stared at the fat girl eating a gooey, chocolate dessert.

There is, by the way, an incredible amount of discrimination against fat people in this country. If you have never been fat, you can't know. The looks on people's faces as they stare . . . The condemnation in their eyes . . . The whispers, whether real or imagined . . . For years before, I was sure other people, especially the skinny ones, were thinking and even saying "No wonder you look like that. I just bet you do that all the time. Ha! Shame on you!"

Now, however, no one stared. No one even looked. There was no guilt. There was no shame. I tried to describe to Mom and Dad (neither of whom have ever been fat) the joyous freedom of eating a completely wicked dessert — guilt-free!

Opportunity is not a carrot dangling just outside your reach. Neither is the new you! You get

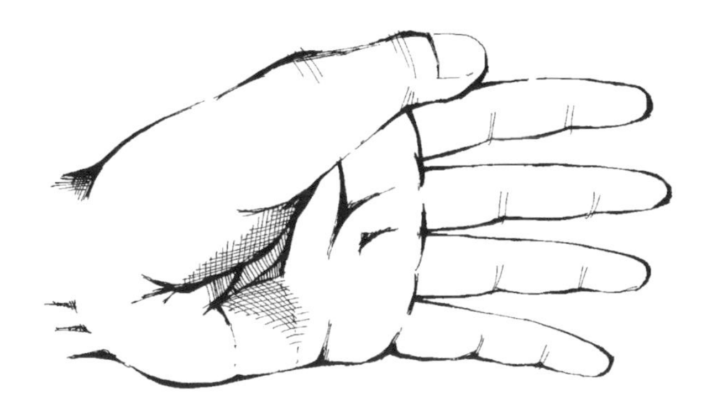

to choose to be different. You can choose health and wealth. You get to choose to remove restrictions and limits. Only you can. Not anyone who loves you. Not anyone who works with you. Not your kids, wife, husband, parent, friend or lover. Only you.

Be sure you do a huge list on each of the following "Your Turn" pages. What will replace what and when will you be rich? When will things get easier? When will the marriage get better? When will your boss realize what you are worth? When will the kids leave home? When will your employees realize how indispensable you are? When will you have more time? Will you change your life then? Or will you keep repeating the patterns? If you truly want your life to be different, you will begin today. Today is where you live.

**Grab onto the new,
Let go of the old:**

- Nothing of value exists in a vacuum.
- You have to let go of the old ways of doing, being, and thinking for space to exist for the new ways.
- You let go through awareness and choice.
- You grab onto the new with clarity and vision.
- It is easier to grab on than to let go of the familiar.

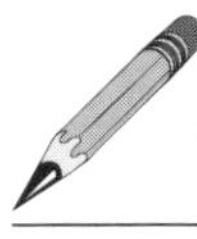

Your Turn

1. What do I need to let go of? (Any ways of doing, being or living.)

2. If I'm not ready to let go, what do I need to do to get willing to let go?

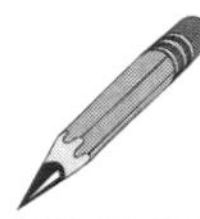

Your Turn

3. What would I like to grab on to in my life to replace each thing I let go of?

Live one day at a time
and make it a masterpiece.

To wish to be well is a part
of becoming well.

— Seneca

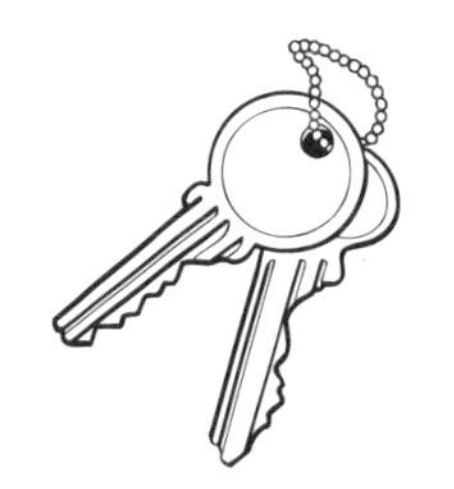

Key # 6:

Embrace a New Way

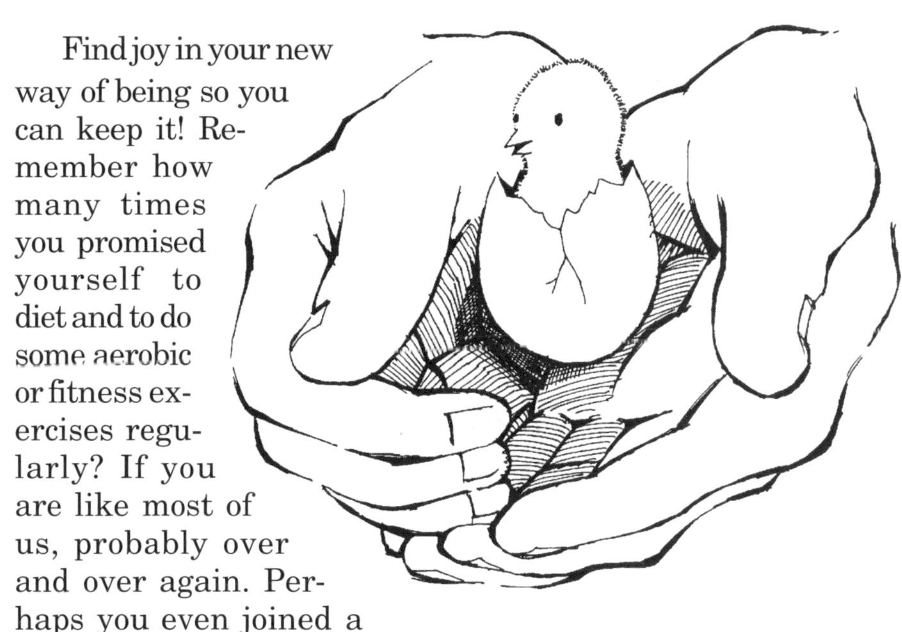

Find joy in your new way of being so you can keep it! Remember how many times you promised yourself to diet and to do some aerobic or fitness exercises regularly? If you are like most of us, probably over and over again. Perhaps you even joined a health club, thinking that a monetary investment would inspire you to work out regularly. Did it?

The only people I know who have stayed with a fitness regime are the ones who discovered an activity or two that they are passionate about. One friend truly enjoys running. Indeed, he needs it. He has become positively addicted to the pleasure he gets from it.

No one can decide for you what inspires you. Figure out what you enjoy, then do it. Your initial effort will then grow into a "must do" activity and lifetime commitment. Be sure to select a new behavior that is fun! It seems to be hard for many of us to have fun regularly, predictably, planned. It's a lot easier to work.

Frequently after a seminar, a client will ask me how to determine what he or she really wants and enjoys in life. I ask, "What do you really love to do?" The client looks at me like I'm crazy! I estimate that 90% of the people I know have never asked themselves this question. We discover our joy when we stop to ask ourselves what brings us joy!

Joy is gladness, delight, exultation, rapture, satisfaction. Do you have it? Are you full of joy? You deserve it. Daily! Now. Don't wait for someone else to provide your joy. You must fill yourself. Only when you are full do you have something to share. First, find it! What brings you joy?

What brings me joy? I absolutely love helping people with small businesses to plan and succeed, working with them to improve their teams and communications. Also, public speaking, writing, recording, scuba diving, hiking, walking, biking, four-wheel exploring, seeking out ghost towns. There's more: travel to faraway places, other cultures, cooking, time with friends, photography, movies, old movies on TV, reading. I love to do more things than I am probably ever going to be able to do in this lifetime.

I am learning to play with children more all the time: blowing bubbles, watching a Slinky work its way down the stairs, playing jacks, being silly, having fun! Children inherently know joy. Unfortunately, we quickly teach them how to be serious. How sad. Such nonsense. When they grow up, they have to relearn joy. Just like us. Let us live and teach balance.

If you don't have what you want,
you are not committed to it 100%.

— Dr. Robert Anthony

How do you figure out what you really love to do?

Close yourself up in a room away from the distractions of the world. Unplug the telephones. If the doorbell rings, ignore it. Ensure no interruptions. You really can, you know! The world won't stop. Light candles or build a fire in the fireplace. Put on relaxing music. Set the stage for your "quiet mind" to work. Gather crayons, markers, or colored pencils and a large pad of paper. Then draw whatever comes to your mind and through your fingers.

Ask yourself over and over: "What do I really love to do? What brings me joy?" For at least an hour keep asking yourself what brings you true joy. Then draw it! Do no writing. Do not analyze or judge your ideas. Just brainstorm. Keep drawing.

At the end of the hour, analyze what you drew. Look at the patterns. Now examine and organize the images. What do the patterns, shapes, designs, colors tell you about yourself? What feelings and memories do they stir? Have you rediscovered a hobby you can turn into an income? If you drew lots of fish — can you fish for a living? Can you buy a boat and crew? Can you open a fish market? Can you cook fish for a living?

I first did this technique after I sold my physical therapy practice. I had sold my old house and was living in a rented townhouse while my new home was being built. I had an incredible view of the foothills to the great Rocky Mountains. This introspective time helped me greatly to determine how I wanted to spend the rest of my life.

IQ tests don't necessarily show our genius. My friend, Paul, is a genius. He knows it and I know it. He has one rule for life: If it isn't fun, he doesn't do it. This is true of his job, his family relationships and friendships, and the theater. I believe he lives one of the most joyful lives of anyone I know. He pays to have his clothes washed, because it isn't fun and he feels he could be doing things much more fun and creative with that time.

For a living, he develops market-timing software for investment funds. Paul is more than a little successful — financially as well as personally. To him, his work is fun! Paul sees himself as a citizen of the universe. He doesn't live in one place too long. He wants to experience the whole planet to the largest extent possible. He has remodeled his life many times.

Paul came into my life when he was given a set of my audio tapes by a mutual friend. He was so impressed with "Management by 100% Responsibility," that he called me. We've been friends ever since.

Paul does not believe in "can't . . . won't . . . it-can't-be-done." He doesn't live in the negative and never will. Paul has generously allowed me to share with you his process for deciding what he loves to do, what brings him joy, and what he will do next:

Six steps to getting "un-stuck," to moving forward to determining what you want to do:

1. First, **ask yourself the most important question you need to decide now,** for example: What should I do with my career, my marriage, my finances, etc.?

2. **Green light sessions:** Spend 30 minutes several times over several days. No judgment is allowed. No "what I think I want." No "what I think I can." Write as many responses to your focus question as fast as you can (themes, bizarre, funny, serious, hard, easy, dangerous). Be creative!

3. **Priority session:** In a 30-minute session, list your priorities, roughly in order. These are your deeply-felt priorities — not what you believe you should do, think and feel. Ask yourself: "What are my 3-6 most important life priorities?"

4. **Highlight session:** In a 30-minute session, highlight, star, circle, or underline which priorities feel like what you want to do with no concerns at the moment as to how you would do them.

5. **Visualization sessions:** Visualize one role per day. Actually imagine yourself in each potential role/position/activity. How do you feel? What does the role look like? Where are you in the image? What are you doing? Be in the picture, still not concerned with how.

   Another visualization: Envision actually attracting all the circumstances or situations that will make your focused desire happen. Now you begin to explore how.

6. **Conclusion:** After this process, you are much more prepared and able to make the decisions necessary to go out and create your new future!

Embrace a new way:

- Finding what brings us joy takes thoughtful action.
- Embrace means encircle, enclose, hug, hold close.
- Joy means glad, delighted, happy.
- We must embrace or find joy in a new way or we will not persist.
- We all deserve joy every day of our lives.

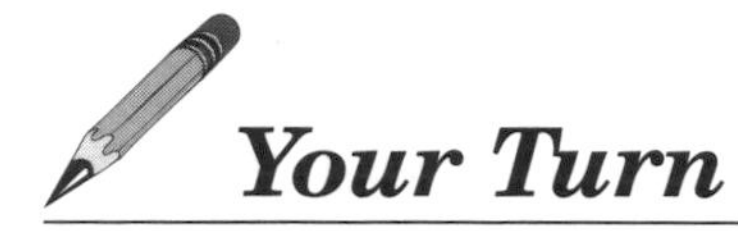

Your Turn

1. What did you discover when you did the exercises above for discovering your joy or your passion? If you haven't done them yet, why not? What's your plan to take the first step? What are you waiting for?

2. What 20 activities, people, things or practices truly make me happy or bring me joy? *Write quickly and without censoring or criticizing your list. Keep going over 20 — we've left room on the next page too.*

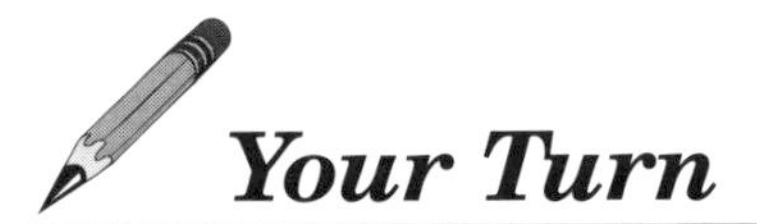

Your Turn

3. Am I doing these things now? If not, why not? Here's my plan to start today.

Many strokes, though with a little axe,
Hew down and fell the hardest-
timber'd oak.

— Shakespeare

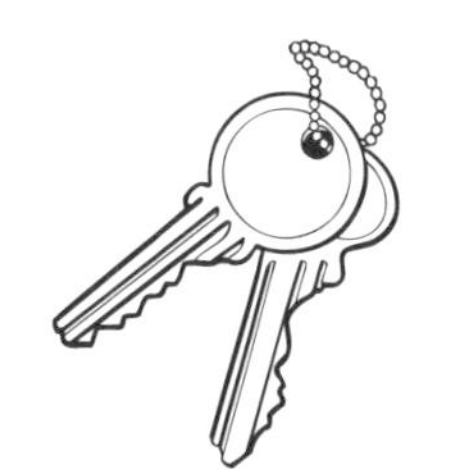

Key # 7:

Stop Playing Victim

I don't believe there are truly any victims on the planet. Some people do grow up being victimized. Some grow up without privileges and comfort. Others live in poverty or where there is war, disease, oppression, and no food. Many people live in horrible conditions. But you know what? Some of those people leave their circumstances. They are not victims. They make choices.

People choose to be victimized; they play victim to their pasts and to their circumstances. It doesn't have to be that way. Generally, people do not consciously or intentionally choose their unhappy lives; certainly children don't. Positive changes in our lives are conscious decisions not to play victim. We must take conscious action to change our lives for the better by making non-victim decisions.

How do mentally and spiritually healthy individuals handle their abusive pasts or victimizations?

- They stop denial.
- They acknowledge the reality of their situations.
- They feel their feelings.
- They deal, then they heal.
- They forgive the perpetrator(s).

You don't have to remain in a position where anyone is hurting you now. If you truly are or were underprivileged, abused, used, victimized, you can change today. Continued obsession about your past mistreatment is victimizing yourself and giving the victimizer continued power over you.

You cannot change the past. You cannot "do" enough guilt to pay for past wrongs or undo them. You can learn from the past and choose not to repeat it. No one is continuing the victimization today but you. No matter how much you blame your parents, spouse, teacher, the marines, the war — or whatever is your particular scapegoat — get help if you need it. Deal with it.

How you live in this present moment is a choice. Guilt will not help. It cannot and does not change anything. Guilt only makes you feel worse. In my seminars, I draw the following graphic to demonstrate past, present and future:

	Past	Present	Future
Body:		X	
Mind:	X		
	Usual here: ~~GUILT~~ Better to: LEARN		

Your body is firmly planted in the present, attending the seminar. I can see, smell, touch and feel to prove that your body is here in the present. Your mind, however, can go anywhere it wants and may very well go back to yesterday, last year, even many years ago. The elderly often mentally go back many years to pleasant memories when their spouse was alive and their body free of pain. Certainly, memories are great; in fact, crucial to mental health. However, as Louise Hay says in her book "You Can Heal Your Life," the point of power is always in the present moment. Only in this moment do we truly live. And only in this moment can we change or deal with past injustices.

You may be bodily present at a seminar but thinking about yesterday's happenings, or what happened ten years ago, or what your spouse said this morning at breakfast. You may feel guilt over real or imagined harms.

I ask seminar participants if they have ever been able to "do" enough guilt to change their past actions and poor choices. They smile, admitting they have not. Certainly, we can't change what was done to us. But the real question is, "What should you do with your past — ignore it?" No. But neither is it helpful to feel guilty or angry. From today forward you can use what you learned from your past to create positive change.

Guilt is a choice. If you did harm to someone, clean up the past by apologizing. Making amends. Paying back. In some significant way take responsibility for causing another person pain.

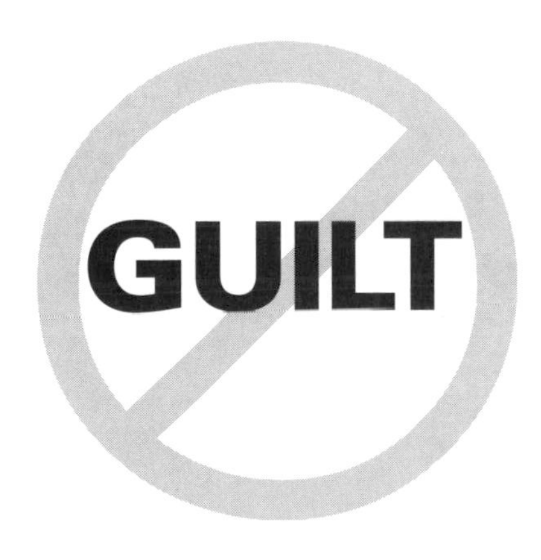

Webster's Dictionary defines guilt as blame, fault, culpability. Guilt often involves shame, too. Shame is only a feeling but it is also a choice.

Have you ever analyzed feelings and thoughts? Webster defines feelings as sensation, an emotion. Can someone else make you feel anything? No. Your feelings are uniquely your own based upon your individual beliefs, experiences and values. Your feelings can only come from your thoughts.

Where, then, do thoughts come from? Can anyone outside you make you think certain thoughts? No. During a seminar each person "hears" the same words but may understand them differently. Guilt is a feeling based on chosen thoughts. You can change your thoughts and, thus, your feelings. No one else can do that for you. You alone have the power to change both your own thoughts and feelings.

There is no absolute truth. Many people may happen to agree with me based upon their own set of beliefs, experiences, and values. Therefore, all the seminar participants hear exactly what they came to hear. And they all hear their own truth — if they are looking for it.

If you were hurt by someone, your only options for joy are: Feel the pain. Deal with it. Let yourself heal. To be free to move on, you also must forgive.

How do you forgive? When your anger is justified and you want to hold it and cherish it forever, how do you forgive someone else's hurtful action toward you?

Start with willingness to forgive.

I agree with Louise Hay when she tells us: "Choose to release the past and forgive everyone, yourself included. You may not know how to forgive. You may not want to forgive. However, being willing to forgive starts your healing process." Here is an affirmation to set you free:

I forgive myself for not being the person I want to be.

I forgive others, and set myself free.

Create your own affirmation for forgiveness to begin healing.

Forgiveness frees you to learn from your past. When you have learned your life lessons, you stop playing victim and you do not repeat your past patterns.

What about the future? With your body in the present, your mind in the future is doing what? Frequently, worrying. My dear grandmother worries about me flying so much and traveling alone. She means, "I love you very much and have great concern for your safety."

I tell her, "If you're going to worry, don't pray. If you're going to pray, don't worry." Can she worry enough to keep me from dying in a plane crash? Can I worry sufficiently to prevent a natural disaster or the death of a loved one? Worry looks like this:

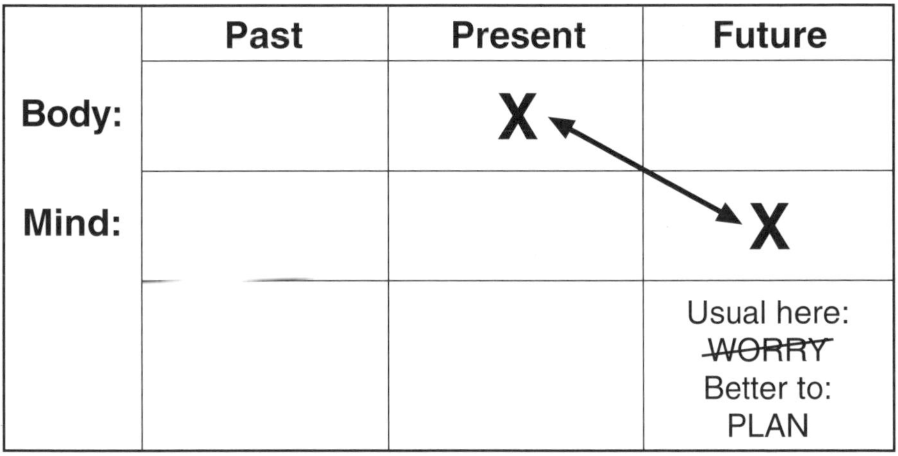

	Past	Present	Future
Body:		X	
Mind:			X
			Usual here: ~~WORRY~~ Better to: PLAN

Worry is like guilt — totally unproductive. Worry doesn't change anything. Worry cannot alter the future, any more than guilt can alter the past. So like the song says, "Don't Worry, Be Happy!" Being happy really is a choice, as is worry a choice.

Use what you can learn from your past to plan your future. We are not able to control all factors, but when we utilize our experiences, including our mistakes, we give up blame and shame and plan ahead to the best of our ability. Planning works when you do the footwork and leave the results to God, or whatever Source you believe in.

When you're attending a seminar or church or a meeting, you may worry about the future or just ahead to tonight: Did I remember to take the fish out of the freezer? What movie will we watch? Will my spouse remember to pick up the kids? What about the ball game? Can we pay the rent tomorrow? It isn't significant how far your mind goes into the future, except that when your mind wanders, you leave the present. And the present is the only time-frame you can change and in which you literally live. Living in the present moment is where all the power for change is.

	Past	**Present**	**Future**
Body:		**X** ↕	
Mind:		**X**	

There are risks in the present. When you truly live here, you have to address what is real right now. Life is scary here and can be very uncomfortable. You are vulnerable in the present. It is in the present that you quit blaming your spouse for all his or her shortcomings. When s/he asks: "What is the problem right now?" you must not address the last ten years, (archeological problem solving) but literally right now.

It takes discipline to keep your thoughts in the present. But, the present is also where all good experiences happen:

- great art
- good music
- true intimacy
- rich friendships
- spiritual experiences
- nature experiences
- good feelings
- all feelings
- love
- creativity

Suppose you die in a car crash tonight? Have you been here and now in each moment of today? Time is the same for all of us. We all have all there is: 24 hours each day. Wishing for more time is futile. The only time any of us has is now. We can only exist in the present moment. So, if you want to change your life, start with this single moment in time.

One of my first incredibly powerful realizations of "present moment" living came after my father was seriously burned. I went to Cozumel, Mexico to be certified for open water diving. I had just mastered neutral buoyancy, a state wherein I didn't float to the surface nor sink in the sand; I just floated perfectly level, not touching anything.

Soon after certification, I was diving close to the ocean floor. The water was clear azure blue, like a Colorado sky in the autumn. Visibility was about 150 feet. The sand was as white as pure sugar. All colors were intensified and my senses were greatly heightened.

I looked up toward the sky through the water. Long, sparkling, gold streams of sunlight shot through the water. A large school of angel fish swam by, in perfect precision, right through the golden fall of light. I was physically and emotionally struck by the beauty. "This is the only moment I have," I realized with shock. I remember thinking "I must memorize every detail so I can re-create it for Dad and take it back to him!"

I was in the present moment. It was the only place I could be — in that time — both physically and mentally.

Nothing even just five minutes past had any real significance. In that sense, the past did not exist. I was captivated by the singular moment. What would happen next would also enthrall me — then.

Floating in the sea, in this moment was my reality. It was all. I could not think ahead to what would happen when I returned to the surface, the boat above, or when I returned home. I knew that in those moments I would be fully there. I would be fully present wherever I was. My life became joyful, vivid, and real!

Another exquisite "present moment" came when one summer I has hiking to the top of a mystical, magical mountain close to Aspen, Mt. Sopris. Twin summits rise to 13,000 feet. My long-legged companion, Don, was climbing over huge, sharp boulders with great ease, unlike the way I enthusiastically squirreled over those boulders with my short legs — four times his steps and strides. I think I must have been an Indian who lived on that mountain in another life. When I go to Glenwood Springs, I always spend some time looking at and meditating upon Mt. Sopris, watching the sunsets turn the great monolith bright pink.

As my friend and I hiked up the mountain, a summer thunderstorm turned intense.

> *Numerous hikers ahead of us were turning around. I had no intention of turning back — short of a life-threatening situation; we had backpacked in to camp at Dinkle Lake at the base of the peaks. We watched the storm come down the valley from McClure Pass, past Redstone to Glenwood, then turn around the mountain and head up toward Aspen. It was awe-inspiring!*
>
> *When we reached the second summit, we looked down on the town of Redstone. Crimson-colored stone cascaded all the way down the mountain. The grass was as green and soft as any putting green. The sky was cobalt. Huge, fluffy, white post-storm clouds spread across the horizon. My heart stopped still! "This is perfect!" I declared into the vast open space. "This is as good as I ever need for life to be!"*

The moment was exultant. I was totally in the present moment. The all-encompassing sensation was mental, physical, spiritual, and emotional. Full value! This was real intimacy with life. Full joy. This moment was worth all the discipline and awareness it took me to make the decision to "Be here now!"

Another "present moment" experience was at a Yanni concert with a young friend, Barb, just graduating from college. She was newly sober and had never been to a concert in that condition. The concert was at the stunning Red Rocks Amphitheater in the foothills just west of Denver. We sat in fresh air, surrounded by giant red rocks, the setting sun turning them a glowing crimson. Yanni's piano concertos lifted us. My miracle moment was watching my young friend's face light up and open up as she truly experienced the music. We both were totally there in the moment. There was no place else to be.

I want my life to always be so simple and uncomplicated as those wonderful experiences. It was also simple and uncluttered that summer of 1980 when I medically demanded and emotionally dictated complete removal from the usual day-to-day life of Colorado. I had to be away from the distractions and obligations of work, house and spouse. My only job was to exercise every day, go to the market and buy, then eat, the best possible food. For transportation, I rode the bike everywhere or relied on my trusty running shoes.

Running on the sand seemed like the ultimate new experience to a Coloradan, and so I did. I developed terrible blisters! One day I went into the running shop and the employees started laughing when I mentioned the miserable blisters. They asked me where I was from. They said, "I bet you're running on the sand, huh?"

I said "Of course. Why not?" The shop personnel assured me that if I would run on a more firm surface, there would be less friction and the blisters would go away. Sure enough, they were right.

The rest of my time was spent listening to how other winners were learning to live life. There was also a lot of time to sit quietly by the ocean. San Diego and Coronado offer sailing, scenery and fantastic things to do. On the beach near the old Hotel Del Coronado, there were abundant birds, shells and rock barriers in the ocean. I was in seventh heaven.

> *There was a slight earthquake while I was there. I was on the telephone with my husband when it hit and I was freaking out. He said "Get under the bed!"*
>
> *I shouted back, "There are about three inches under the bed. No way I can fit!"*
>
> *He said, "Go stand in the doorway." The doorway was weaving and dancing all over the place, like a drunken sailor. If I stood in the doorway I would fall out of the building. Glasses were falling in the sink and crashing out of cupboards.*

> *But afterwards, the beach was instantly transformed into a brand new, ethereal landscape. Rocks appeared which weren't there before. Sand disappeared. The beach grew, then shrunk again like something dried in too hot a clothes dryer. Nothing fit. All the shells were different. The waves were even different; bigger, wilder, less predictable. The birds were disoriented. But the sunsets stayed the same. All pink and gold, with a sometimes sharp and dark, sometimes blurry, foggy outline of Point Loma and Cabrillo National Monument, across the water to the west.*

It was like being a kid again! Yes, life can be that clear and simple again. It is my choice.

I met lots of wonderful people and made a few new friends. But, mostly, I learned to just spend time with me. I had been married and surrounded by so many people for so long, learning to just get along with me, healthy, was quite a new experience. Part of the experience was the growing and expanding awareness of how much I had, how fortunate and indeed blessed I was.

More recently, I was privileged to share another intensely spiritual present moment experience with my friend, Connie.

> *It is the most beautiful lake I have ever seen. Much as I hate to admit, it may be even more breathtaking than Colorado's own Fern Lake or Lake Agnes. It was nine o'clock on a long summer evening way to the north of us. The sun was only beginning to set, and that heavy, warm, golden glow was wrapping itself around the surrounding peaks. All the colors were indescribably bright, vivid and clear.*

This is Moraine Lake and it is in the beyond-spectacular Rocky Mountains of Alberta, Canada, about ten miles south of the village of Lake Louise. This magical looking glass sits in the Valley of the Ten Peaks. High, rugged peaks, pure white clouds, trees, snow, and shale were so perfectly reflected in the water, that on the developed photos most people turn the photo upside down because the image is even more blue and clear than the sky.

Connie and I had just finished dinner and decided to hike into bear country. The crowds had begun to thin late in the evening, and there were signs all around us declaring that bear had been seen on that very trail in the last few days. Connie was dying to see bear! She kept asking "What are we going to do if we see one? Gee, I hope we see one!"

As the great authority I am on bears, I assured her that what we would do was stand our ground, never run, walk with big sticks, and if worse came to worse, and one charged us we would just cram our cameras down its throat. Then it couldn't eat us! I looked at her and realized she had this little, tiny point-and-shoot type of camera. It would not even have served as an appetizer.

There were flocks of tiny, duck-like birds which suddenly disappeared straight down into the water, all at once — as though somebody gave a secret signal. We could clearly see every rock under the water. Logs were floating everywhere. The smell was heavy, cool, rich, loamy. We could see fish and little eddies under the water. There were bubbles coming out from under some of the rocks, perhaps from a bubbling spring.

We laughed. And we hiked. And we talked. But, the best was when we just sat in silence and felt it all. When we looked at all of nature perfectly mirrored in that incredible, amazing blue water. It was a feeling of completeness; of this is it! A knowing that there is not another place on the planet I would rather be in this one perfect moment.

Living in the present moment takes discipline and desire. We can only embrace a new way in this moment. We cannot find joy in any moment but the one we are in. It doesn't exist in the past nor in the future. We stop playing victim and leave the past behind — in the present moment.

Once we have gained the ability to live in the present moment, we are prepared to offer this gift to others. We are ready to serve others. We are assured of continued high quality present moments by surrounding ourselves with positive, supportive people who share our dreams with us.

Stop playing victim:

- If you truly have been victimized, stop letting the perpetrator victimize you now.
- Make a decision to be a non-victim now.
- Forgive the abuser or victimizer.
- Learn to leave the past in the past, let the future be in the future.
- Choose to live in the present moment.
- Choose all your feelings and thoughts.

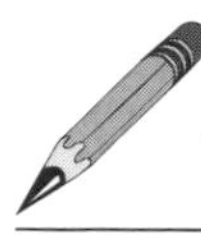

Your Turn

1. Who do I need to forgive? Do I need to forgive me? Do I need to forgive me for not being perfect?

2. Am I still being a victim of anything current or past? If so, why am I still allowing myself to be victimized? What's my first step to stop?

There is no denying that most of us, when we arrive at a place, immediately begin to think of other places to which we may go from it.

— Mercelene Cox

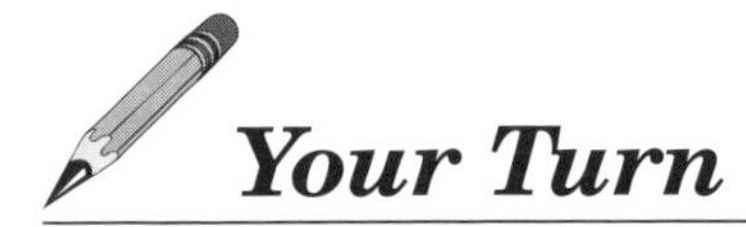

Your Turn

3. Here's how I know I am living in the present moment.

Every good thought you think is contributing its share to the ultimate result of your life.

— *Anonymous*

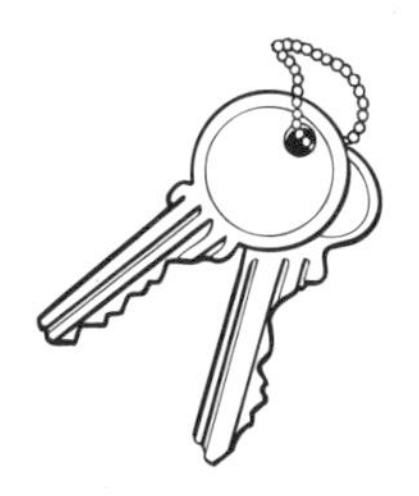

Serve Others

What good is "self-improvement," "self-help," "changing self" if it is only self-serving? Frequently, those of us wishing to change something in our lives either have no boundaries and are too eager to people-please to be healthy — or we are very self-centered.

A friend, Jerry, whom I very much admire, noted that the problem with self-help books and many motivational speakers is that they are all about self: What can I get for me? What will this do for me? How can I improve my life, finances, relationships, et al? "They are too self-centered," Jerry said. "Without a willingness to share the good, and spend time, energy and resources in service to others, isn't it all meaningless? Isn't it all just so much empty talk?" Good sense, my friend.

Every great religion, philosophy, theory, belief system, and spiritual teacher I have studied has, in some way, emphasized service. Commonalities in these beliefs are the basic principles of love, honesty, integrity, acceptance, faith, trust, courage, humility, forgiveness, surrender, willingness, freedom, perseverance, patience, and service.

If we don't commit to service, we find ourselves locked into dark and dangerous places. When we reach out and find service that suits us and our personalities, we find our unique place and abilities in society. We are privileged to give back some of what has been freely given to us.

I have sought my niche over many years and have found it in legion hours of volunteered time to people recovering from addictions: phone time, personal time, meals prepared, overnights provided. I am privileged to see miracles happen: people getting productive, love-filled lives back.

My friend, Cia, spends time at a public broadcasting station seeking financial support for quality television. She also rides in the "Courage Classic," a 150-mile bicycle ride to collect pledges for Children's Hospital. She does not have to do this. She could just donate money. She enjoys giving her time and personal commitments to the causes in which she believes.

Deborah used to spend five hours a week helping at a "halfway house" for women still serving time out of prison. Most of them have committed three or more felonies. Some of them are drug addicts, some alcoholics, some drug dealers, and others have committed crimes of various types for which they are learning to take responsibility.

Deb's motivation flowed from deep gratitude that her own addictions led her close to prison herself. Only by grace and sobriety was she spared. The service work gratified her because she got to be a part of people's learning new life skills in a practical and responsible manner. I knew Deb for over a year before she even told me she gave this time in service.

Some of my family members have gone to Africa, Tibet, and China as missionaries. My parents, more than ten years after leaving Rwanda, still send money to support children in the schools there and to help feed the little ones caught up in the political chaos.

Many of my friends don't tell what they do to be of service because telling might be for self-glorification. Humility and private sharing are more of value to them.

Do you give some time to others in service? Do you volunteer?

If you haven't considered some positive action to make a difference, you might want to write down some interests or causes you believe in and could work for to say thank-you for all the good in your life. Gratitude is attitude plus action.

There are many ways we can make a difference in people's lives. We can serve in professional capacities as well as personal and spiritual. I know that I am meant to serve. I give to the power of good on the planet through speaking, training, books, audio tapes, consulting, volunteering, serving on boards of directors or anything else that shows up! Beauty, hope and love are to be shared and they've been so freely given to me and to you!

Serve Others:

- Service is important because it takes us out of "self."
- It makes us feel good about giving back.
- It creates positive feelings and good results on the planet.
- It actually can make a significant difference in someone's life and future.

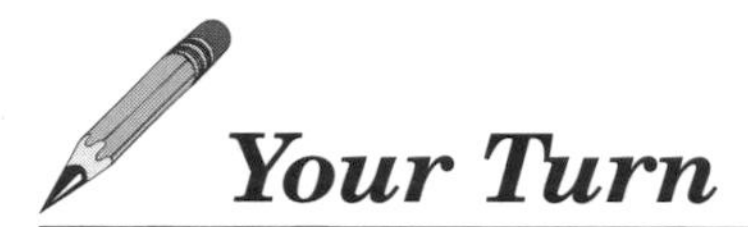

Your Turn

1. What does service really mean to me?

2. What/where can I do some service for others at least weekly?

Every action of our lives touches on some chord that will vibrate in eternity.

— Edwin Hubbel Chapin

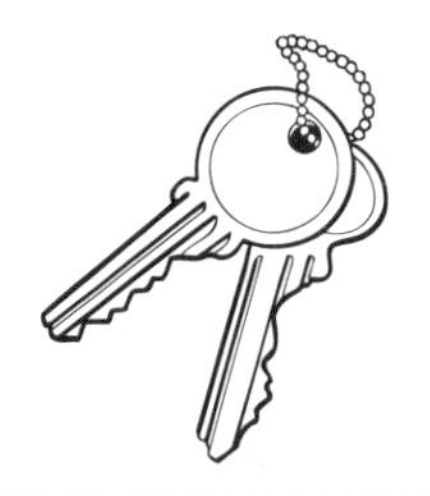

Surround Yourself with Positive, Supportive People Who Share Your Dreams!

Choose who to be around — at work, home, play, everywhere. Otherwise, you might not have the encouragement you need from others during your tough times. (You may have less control over this at work. Do the best you can. You can choose your work friends.)

Are you prepared for the tough times? There will be tough times. You already know this. You no doubt have tried to change patterns or behaviors before. Even when our intentions are great, lasting change can be challenging at times. We all need others.

Where do you find supportive people who will help you keep and share your dreams? Maybe they are already in your life? If the people in your family or home do not seem to be on your side or willing to support you, perhaps they do not know you want or need their support.

Be clear with your loved ones and friends about what you need and how you need for them to help you. Ask for what you need. Clearly. Plainly. Directly. This is no time for manipulation or games, such as "He knows I need to be told he loves me, or that I am beautiful, or that he cares or is there for me, or that he wants me to do well." No fair!

Generally, I am straightforward and direct. However, in truly intimate conversations or when I need personal support, I continue to work very hard to be: Clear. Plain. Direct. And to just ask. It works when I am willing. People like to be asked.

If you have not found positive, supportive people in your life, then actively and with clear purpose seek them out. There is so much negativity in our world. It takes effort and active, conscious choosing to find and only associate with positive people. Look for these people in churches, groups, meetings, at work, in support groups and clubs where people share your interests. Think way outside your normal "box!"

Remember my friend Paul and his winning formula for changing directions and discovering what you love to do? Here is Paul's story about how he learned to live his life fully and positively; how he discovered the power of surrounding himself with positive, supportive people who share his dreams:

> *In terms of preparing for a promising career, Paul began life on the wrong foot. Neither of his parents completed high school. His own schooling began in a very low-income ghetto neighborhood. His educational experience was not particularly stimulating. Then he mistook boredom and poor grades for an inability to learn. He dropped out of high school, though eventually he obtained a diploma through an alternative, trade-oriented public school. Paul began his career poorly-educated and essentially illiterate.*
>
> *After several years of disappointing dead-end jobs, a brief tour of military duty, a divorce, and becoming a single parent, Paul had come to accept his lot in life — an unrewarding career with limited financial potential. It was pretty clear to him that he was on a course for continued disappointment in life.*

Fortunately, however, Paul met a person who shared some motivational concepts with him and encouraged him to read short articles and listen to audio tapes by authors like Maxwell Maltz, W. Clement Stone, and Earl Nightingale. Though these new ideas were inspiring to Paul, it was difficult for him to believe they would work for him. After all, he had a very poor education and limited job skills. Nonetheless, as time went on, Paul came to a point when he said to himself, "What have I got to lose? Maybe, just maybe, I could learn to choose differently for my future. Maybe I am playing victim, letting my past be an excuse for not going anywhere in the present."

The thought of a new life and a bright future was intriguing and compelling to Paul, but he was still guarded since he had never experienced success. So he decided to put these new motivational concepts to the test. He enrolled in a night class at the local junior college. Instead of just taking the class, however, he threw himself into it. After all, if he just muddled through, that would prove nothing and the class would be a complete waste of his time.

Paul decided not to focus on the exam scores or the final grade. Rather he decided to make the experience as fun and exciting as possible. He could not imagine being able to persist in this class if it were as painful and unrewarding as high school. The test would, once and for all, prove or disprove the merit of all these hypothetical motivational concepts he'd been reading about. If the concepts proved to be

> *false, then Paul would go on with his life as usual. A few weeks of his spare time were all that he would lose.*
>
> *At first, the course work seemed impossible. All the other students seemed much smarter and better prepared. The homework was difficult. The first exam scores were disappointing. At times Paul felt like giving up. But he decided to see this test through to the end. So, night after night he persisted. He attended every class, handed in every homework assignment, read all the materials and studied for every exam. Frequently Paul stayed after class to talk with the instructor and ask questions.*
>
> *As the weeks wore on, the material slowly began to make sense. Paul was able to contribute to class discussions and actually did well on the midterm exam. One success led to another and in the end, he received the highest score in the class on the final exam and an A for the course. More importantly, Paul discovered that his former self-image as a victim of his past experiences and the belief that he was doomed to repeat those experiences was absolutely false. He could indeed learn and it was very rewarding.*
>
> *By the time Paul had finished this class, he had become "addicted" to motivational books and audio tapes. He continued to learn and apply what he learned. He began trying to imagine his future possibilities. What would he do with his newfound knowledge?*

Soon, an old dream started coming back to him, an "impossible" dream that he'd had many years before. As a child frequently Paul pretended he was a great engineer or scientist, but that dream had died, as he became more and more discouraged with life in general and school in particular. But now maybe, just maybe, his dream was possible. Did he dare to believe that he could make it through college? The thought both excited and frightened him.

At this point Paul was about to learn the most valuable lesson of his life. In attempting to follow his dream he felt very vulnerable. He was a prime target for every nay-sayer in the universe. They seemed to crawl out of the woodwork and enjoy giving him the "benefit" of all their great wisdom.

The nay-sayers were well meaning. They probably did not consciously know the damage they did. They thought they were giving Paul some great advice "for his own good." The most devastating nay-sayers were his family members, trusted friends, and those in-places-of-authority-and-thus-know-these-things and to question their opinion was heresy.

The nay-sayers told Paul all the reasons why he could not possibly accomplish his goal. They pointed out how naive he was to even consider such an undertaking. "Do you know what you are getting yourself into?" they asked. "I've seen people try that one before, and they fell right on their faces!" They went on to point out every little "fact" that supported their assessments. "You are too old, young, fat, skinny. You're not the right gender or race. You don't have the right looks, aptitude, personality, background, training, credentials." And on and on. Worse yet, the nay-sayer's "facts" were very often true.

When Paul announced that he was going to go to engineering school, his boss said, "After all we've done for you here at the company, and this is how you repay us? Hey, this is a company on the move. If you leave now, you'll regret it. We'll have to replace you and there is no way you can get your old job back. This is the biggest mistake of your entire life."

Of course his most helpful friend said, "There is no way that a single parent can afford child-care without a full-time job. You are being selfish. You've got to think of your daughter." Another friend just laughed and said "You, go to college? Yeah, right!"

The most devastating nay-sayer was the Admissions Counselor at the university who pointed out several "facts" that were hard to deny. "Paul, I've got to tell it to you straight. We turn away thousands of applicants who have B averages, and you graduated in the bottom ten percent of your class. My hands are tied. I simply cannot approve your application, then deny someone else who has a much better scholastic record. Let's be realistic. The students who get into our engineering school are at the top of their classes. They've been through all the college prep classes, calculus, physics, and chemistry. You haven't even had trigonometry, let alone science classes. Other than the one junior college class, you haven't had any formal education for quite some time. Our freshman engineering students have been preparing for years for engineering school; even then, 25 percent of them won't make it through their freshman year. With your background, how can you possibly keep up?

Then there is the problem of your financial aid. You've saved enough for the first semester's tuition and books; but neither you nor your parents have the necessary financial capability

> *beyond that. With your high school record, institutional financial aid is simply out of the question. I am sorry to be so direct, but it would be unfair of me to get your hopes up."*
>
> *Paul made one last desperate attempt by asking, "Isn't there some way I could get into this university, even on a part-time basis?" The counselor replied, "Absolutely not. Not as a student anyway. Paul, let me be blunt. The only way you could get into this university would be to apply for a janitor's position!"*

And so Paul's dream died. The counselor's "facts" were irrefutable. Perhaps his boss and friends had been right also. At this point Paul began to wonder how he could have been so naive? He hit a brick wall. Obviously he could not go forward. Then again, he soon found he could not simply go back to his old life style either — living one day to the next, with no hope of a brighter future. He had hit bottom. He was angry, depressed and miserable.

> *In desperation, finally Paul decided to put the motivational concepts to the test once again. "Persistence and creativity" the motivational tapes said. "If you can't get through the front door, try the back." Paul decided to plead his case before the Dean of the Engineering School. Instantly he ran into the next nay-sayer — the Dean's secretary. She, too, had all the right "facts." "The Dean is a very busy person with absolutely no spare time. He simply doesn't see any applicants until they have been accepted by admissions."*
>
> *However, after several pleading calls, to Paul's surprise the secretary said the Dean*

would be having lunch in his office that day and if Paul were extremely brief, the dean would listen.

The Dean quietly ate his lunch while Paul gushed out his story non-stop from beginning to end. Paul even told the dean all about the "facts" the Admissions Counselor had told him. Finally, Paul admitted that all the facts everyone had brought to his attention were true; what's more, he didn't know if he could make it through engineering school. However, if there were any exceptions to the rules, he wanted a chance to try, if for no other reason than to prove it to himself.

The Dean let Paul finish his story, then picked up the phone, called the Admissions Counselor and requested that Paul be given a "special student" status. This meant that all Paul's courses would be taken on a "no-credit" basis and he could only enroll in a class if there was space left after everyone else had enrolled. The Dean told Paul his biggest hurdle would be freshman calculus and suggested two remedial math classes to give him the background he needed. He also told Paul that if he maintained a good grade-point average, he could petition the College of Engineering Council to see if they would retroactively accept his past credits and allow him to enroll in a degree program. The Dean warned Paul, "There are no promises, Paul. The Council could deny your petition."

All Paul could say was "Great. Fine. That's OK! All I want is a chance." As Paul left the Dean's office, the Dean winked at him and

> *smiled, saying, "Oh, by the way. I chair the College of Engineering Council, and I'll be expecting that petition. Don't let me down." As Paul left, he didn't remember his feet even touching the floor!*

Paul graduated from engineering school, third in his class, with "Special Honors." Getting this degree was by no means easy. In fact it was even tougher than he had imagined. But it was also the most exciting and thrilling adventure of his entire life. He was elected president of two engineering honorary societies and he started a tutorial program in which top students volunteered their time to help students who were struggling during their freshman years.

Upon graduation, Paul received 13 job offers. The company he joined put him through graduate school at Stanford University, all expenses paid. During his career Paul has founded three high-tech companies, lectured at three universities, and become a millionaire before he was 40.

How did Paul overcome these irrefutable "facts" that his friends and the admissions counselor had so generously brought to his attention? He declares that the nay-sayers did not realize that a dream coupled with a burning desire transcends seemingly impenetrable obstacles. Paul created circumstances that would bring his dream into reality. He did not buy into the nay-sayer's arguments — and his dream lives.

I am privileged to know many magnificent, unselfish, spiritually growing human beings. They live the 7 Keys. They choose to change their lives. After hurting enough, they all asked for help and accepted responsibility for their choices. They did not quit. They grabbed onto the new and let go of the old. They no longer play victims. Today, they fully embrace finding joy and bringing joy to others. As a result of putting the 7 Keys into their lives, they are able to serve others. These growing, loving human beings surround themselves with positive, supportive people who share their dreams.

You can, too! If you are inspired to move forward — to create a new life for yourself — do it now. If you wait, your enthusiasm may wane. You may start to doubt. Don't let yourself slip back into all the old ways of doing, being, thinking. Go for it!

Write down your commitment. Call someone and tell him or her what you are going to commit to. Call me and tell me your story. Write down your story. Who knows? You may end up in a sequel. Think about Paul and all the others you and I know who have experienced and indeed been able to create change forever.

Discovering and fulfilling your dreams, creating positive change in your life, is a life's journey. There is no quick fix. Each new concept, experience, understanding builds upon and reinforces those that came before. They all require constant practice and vigilance.

I have come to know that the journey is much more important than the destination. I will choose to continue growing and seeking while I:

Cherish Yesterday,
Dream Tomorrow,
Live Today.

Surround yourself with positive, supportive people who share your dream:

- They may be in your life now.
- Tell them what you need and want to create change.
- Ask for their support.
- Believe and take action.
- Start now — don't put off your changes either large or small.

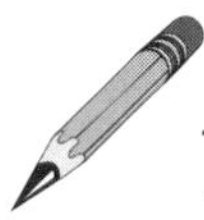

Your Turn

1. Who do I now have in my life who is positive and supportive?

2. How will I tell them how and when I need their support?

Victory belongs to the most persevering.

— Napoleon

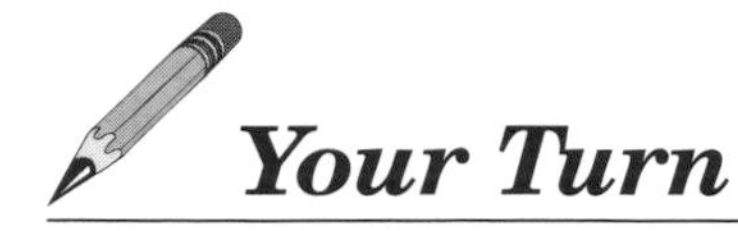

Your Turn

3. Who else would I like to add to this list? Here's how I plan to ask each one.

4. Where and when will I seek new friends and support?

In the long run, men only hit what they aim at.

— Henry David Thoreau

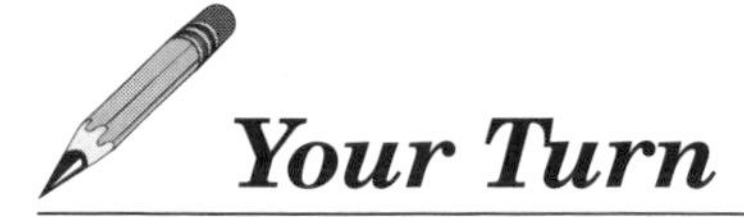

Your Turn

5. Use this space for any other ideas, commitments, action plans — whatever works for you to keep going.

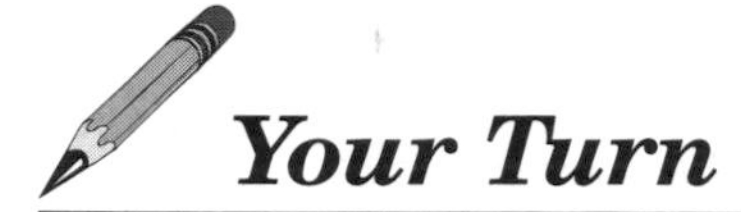

Your Turn

6. Choose a "progress partner" who you can share with on an ongoing basis. Put his/her name and phone number here. Add notes of encouragement, success stories, questions and issues to talk about.

7 Keys to Changing
Your Life, Health and Wealth:

① Choose differently!

This is: "I don't want to continue fat . . . unhappy . . . angry . . . violent . . . drunk . . . being always tardy . . . in hatred . . . perfectionist. This is uncomfortable and I want to move." This decision also involves admitting and acknowledging at some level: "I chose this." Accepting choice is very hard.

② Hurt enough to want to change!

Addicts and former fat people call this "hitting bottom." It applies to all areas where change is needed. It might be thoughts or attempts at suicide, threats of loss of job, family, or anything else you value.

③ Ask for help and accept responsibility for your choices!

I personally have never known anyone to accomplish either small or large changes without being humbled enough to ask for help, then to accept responsibility for doing all it takes to create a new result. Our culture does not support attitudes of responsibility.

④ Never quit!

Negative thoughts and beliefs are such a part of our culture that you must "keep on keeping on" and surround yourself with people and ideas that are positive and inspiring. Faith and trust in your chosen path are also part of not quitting. Many changes are lifestyle and life-long changes.

⑤ Grab onto the new, let go the old!

For change to be real and lasting, you must make a decision, a commitment to let go your old way of thinking, doing, being, living. You can't hold the old and the new at the same time. You must let go of the old for space to exist for the new. Letting go is harder than grabbing on.

⑥ Embrace a new way!

Find JOY in it to persist! It is just like starting an exercise or aerobic program: Find an exercise you truly enjoy to do it enthusiastically for longer than two weeks! You must find something that is fun for you in the long haul.

⑦ Stop playing victim!

No one did this to you — despite how much you want to believe your parents or the past or whatever did it to you. Even if you truly were victimized, today is today and you must decide to leave the past in the past. How? Apply these 7 Keys. Then:

Serve others.
Surround yourself with positive,
Supportive people who
Share your dream!

There is one thing you always
choose . . . your attitude!

There is one thing you always
can change . . . your attitude!

Selected Bibliography

Anthony, R., *Think.* (New York: Berkley Books, 1985.)

Canfield, J. and Hansen, M., *Chicken Soup for the Soul.* (Deerfield Beach, Florida: Health Communications, Inc., 1993.)

Hay, L., *You Can Heal Your Life.* (Santa Monica, California: Hay House, 1987.)

Huston, T. and Rizzo, K., *More Than Mountains: The Todd Huston Story.* (Boise, Idaho: Pacific Press Publishing Association, 1995.)

Stanley, T. and Danko, W., *The Millionaire Next Door.* (Atlanta, Georgia: Longstreet Press, 1998.)

Wholey, D., *The Courage to Change.* (Boston, Massachusetts: Houghton Mifflin Company, 1984.)

Willey, T., *The Power of Choice.* (Denver, Colorado: Berwick House, 1988).

Training and Development Seminars

by Linda McNeil

The following seminars are available for your staff, association, convention or public event:

7 Keys to Change — Four to seven hour course utilizing this book; can be applied in a personal or spiritual arena or in a business setting to deal with imposed change. Up to a full day of interaction, fun, enlightenment and inspiration. If you or your company are ready to deal with change, this course will give you exactly what you need — now!

Dynamite Customer Service — Four to six hour course focuses on the importance of providing excellent customer support. Information for new programs and enhancing current ones is provided in an entertaining and positive way. Tools are given for dealing with the public, telephone etiquette, and communicating with angry and/or difficult clients.

Future Planning — Four to six hour course complete with actual consulting forms for doing your own business strategy and marketing plan in one day. Analyzes business strengths, weaknesses, target markets, and provides ten Keys to planning success.

How to Build Teams and Relationships — Three to six hour course which enhances work relationships and communications by utilizing self-administered, self-interpreted DiSC™ personality profiles, with many interactive exercises. Fun and educational!

If I Can, You Can! — Inspiring keynote address by Ms. McNeil based on the 7 Keys in this book. Great for associations, conferences and retreats.

Linda is a member of the National Speakers Association and the Colorado Speakers Association.

Choices & Changes Unlimited

Call: (303) 277-9488 or 1-800-748-3488
P.O. Box 280234
Lakewood, CO 80228

Internet Addresses:

linmcneil@aol.com
www.vsanet.com/mcneil
www.linmcneil.com

DiSC™ and Other Personality Profiles

Learning to Work Together

by Linda L. McNeil, Team Builder/Consultant/Speaker/Change Coach

The DiSC™ Personal Profile System helps each person learn about his or her own strengths, weaknesses and tendencies under pressure or stress. Understanding ourselves and others helps us to:

- Understand our effect on others
- Appreciate each other's differences
- Adapt strategies to communicate better
- Listen more effectively
- Build better relationships
- Enhance conflict resolution skills
- Improve staff retention
- Improve hiring practices and protocol

DiSC™ is one of the most successful and widely-used personal and professional development tools ever created. It is a self-reporting personality profile from the Carlson Learning Company in Minneapolis, MN, in popular use since 1972. Linda McNeil prefers it to other profiles because of its simplicity and practical applicability.

The four primary descriptive personality types include:

- Dominance
- Influence
- Steadiness
- Conscientiousness

While everyone has every trait, some traits are stronger in each individual. These tendencies determine our behavior as we play and work with others. There is no "right" or "best" characteristic, so there is no need to judge, label, or limit behaviors.

DiSC™ can be administered to individuals or groups by Linda McNeil, who is trained and certified. Lin can also train someone in your company to administer the profile to your employees.

Descriptions of Other Available Products:

Linda McNeil is a public speaker, team builder and consultant who has recorded a number of seminar materials on audio tapes with accompanying textbooks. They are available specific to physical therapy (PT) and other businesses. Please order accordingly. Descriptions of the products follow:

Management by 100% Responsibility — Three powerful 60-minute audio tapes and workbooks dealing with attitudes in the workplace. Featuring real world examples, this is an excellent introduction to management's roles and requirements. Demonstrates how different personalities communicate and tend to deal with stress and change. Incl. handouts and textbook. (appropriate for all) **$49.95**

Dynamite Customer Service — Two entertaining 45-minute audio tapes with textbook that review what it takes to really connect with your customers. Customers will not just be satisfied, but delighted. Includes information for improving front office procedures and telephone etiquette. Incl. textbook. (PT and small business) **$29.95**

Future Planning — Two 40-minute audio tapes with workbook, actual consulting forms and computer diskette for ongoing duplication of forms. This package is designed to lead you through the process of business planning and marketing strategy in a one day do-it-yourself format. 10 Keys for truly successful planning. (PT and small business) **$49.95**

What Does My Staff REALLY Want? — 40-minute audio tape with handout. If you want to better understand staff motivation, this is the tape for you. The ideas were obtained from staff and client interviews over years of employing hundreds of people, followed by ten years of consulting. (PT) **$14.95**

7 Keys to Changing Your Life, Health and Wealth (book) — These 7 Keys will change your life — if you are ready to change your life, health and/or wealth. Be inspired to move forward and enjoy Lin McNeil's personal and professional change experiences! **$12.95**

Order form next page:

Order Form

Name/Title ______________________________

Company ______________________________

Address ______________________________

City ______________ State ________ Zip ________

Phone (   ) ______________________________

Special Offer:

20% OFF when you order at least three products and only one shipping/handling charge of $5.00.

Satisfaction Guaranteed or your money back.

Name of Product	Price	N0.	$S/H	$ Total
Management by 100% R (all)	$49.95		$3.00	$
Future Planning (for PT)	$49.95		$3.00	$
Future Planning (Sm.Bus.)	$49.95		$3.00	$
Dynamite Cust. Serv. (for PT)	$29.95		$3.00	$
Dynamite Cust. Serv. (Sm.Bus.)	$29.95		$3.00	$
What Does My Staff... (for PT)	$14.95		$3.00	$
BOOK: 7 Keys to...(all)	$12.95		$3.00	$
TOTALS:				$

Mail Check Payable to:

Choices & Changes Unlimited
P.O. Box 280234
Lakewood, CO 80228

Or Charge to: Visa ☐ MasterCard ☐

Card Number: ______________________________

Exp. Date: ___/___ Signature as on card: ______________________________

Call to Charge: (303) 277-9488 or 1-800-748-3488

Reader Survey

Open Mind Publishing would greatly appreciate you taking two minutes to complete this reader survey so that we may continue to meet the needs of the reading public:

Please print:

Name/Title ______________________________

Company ______________________________

Address ______________________________

City ______________ State ________ Zip ________

Phone ( ) ______________________________

Did you enjoy the 7 Keys? *(please check one)* ☐ yes ☐ no

Would you purchase another book by this author? ☐ yes ☐ no

Do you frequently purchase self help/inspirational books? ☐ yes ☐ no

Do you frequently purchase inspirational audio tapes? ☐ yes ☐ no

Do you frequently purchase educational audio tapes? ☐ yes ☐ no

Do you frequently purchase business audio tapes? ☐ yes ☐ no

Do you prefer video tapes to audio tapes? ☐ yes ☐ no

What made you decide to purchase 7 Keys?

☐ price ☐ topic ☐ knew author ☐ seminar

Additional comments you would like to make to help us serve you better:

____

____

____

Thank you very much for taking the time to respond to this survey.

Please return survey to: **Open Mind Publishing**
P.O. Box 280234
Lakewood, CO 80228

As a special thank you we will send you a valuable Gift Certificate.
It is our pleasure to serve you!